Selected Topics in Myasthenia Gravis

*Edited by Isam Jaber Al-Zwaini
and Ali AL-Mayahi*

Published in London, United Kingdom

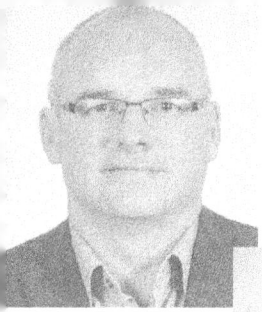
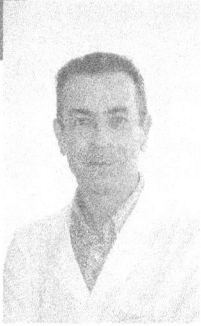
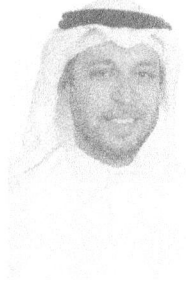
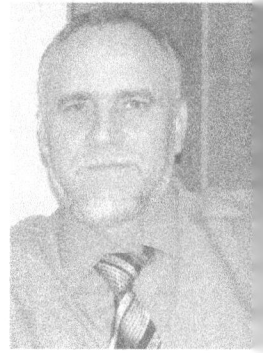
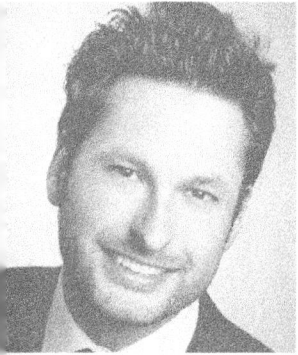
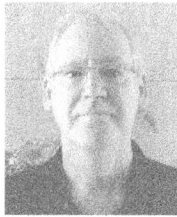
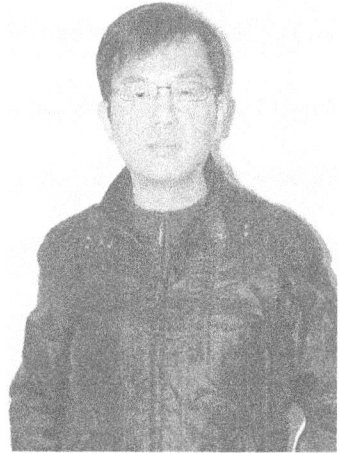

IntechOpen

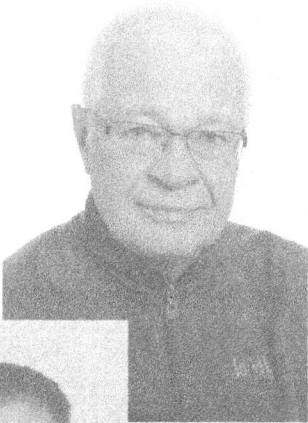
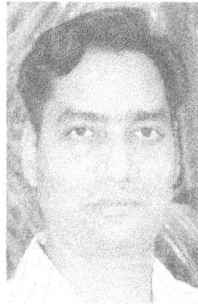
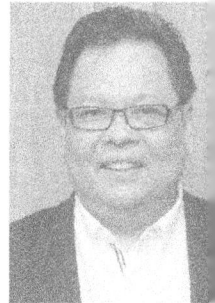
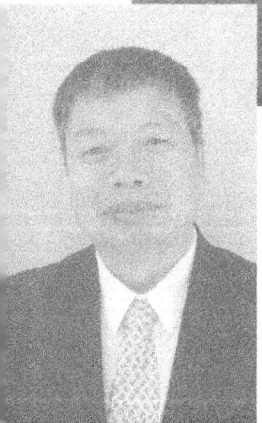
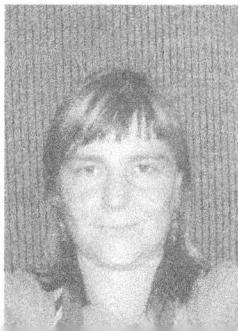
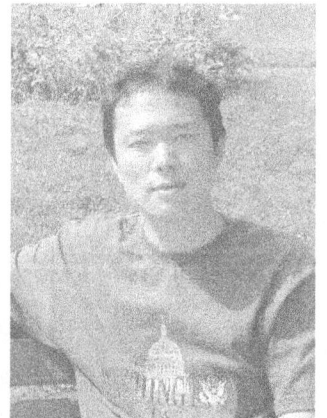

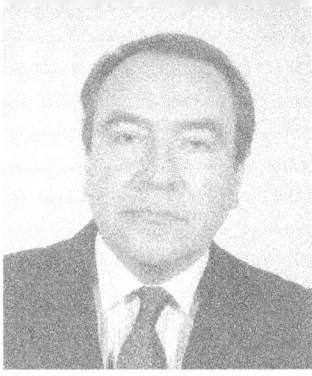

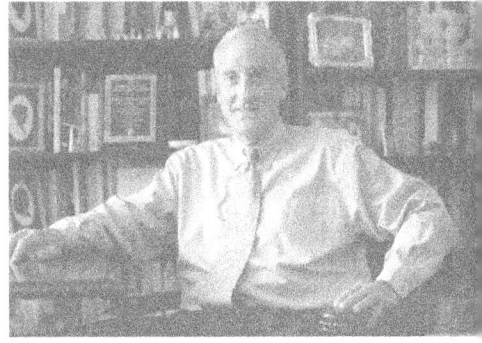

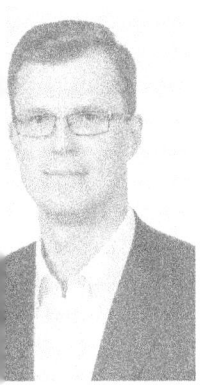

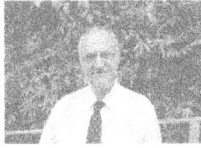

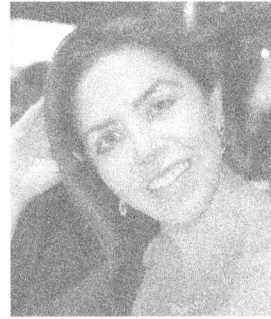

Supporting open minds since 2005

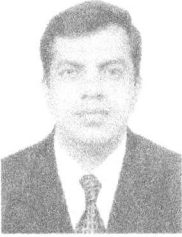

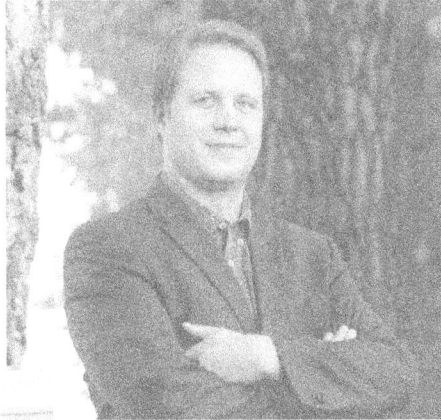

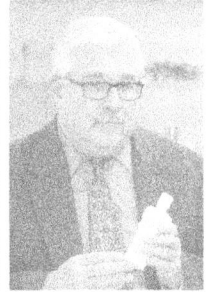

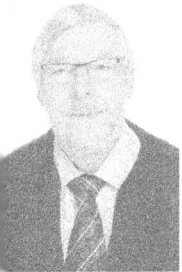

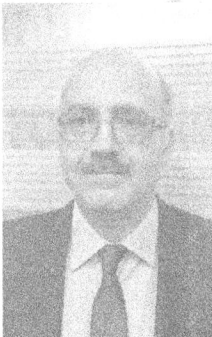

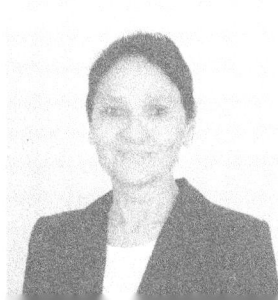

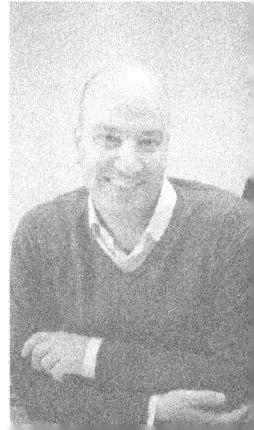

Selected Topics in Myasthenia Gravis
http://dx.doi.org/10.5772/intechopen.73959
Edited by Isam Jaber Al-Zwaini and Ali AL-Mayahi

Contributors
Miljana Z Jovandaric, Svetlana J. Milenkovic, Valerii Voinov, Zeynep Özdemir, Mehmet Abdullah Alagöz, Adel A. Kareem, Lin Chen, Jiang Xu, Kaori Noridomi, Isam Jaber Al-Zwaini

Notice
Statements and opinions expressed in the chapters are these of the individual contributors and not necessarily those of the editors or publisher. No responsibility is accepted for the accuracy of information contained in the published chapters. The publisher assumes no responsibility for any damage or injury to persons or property arising out of the use of any materials, instructions, methods or ideas contained in the book.

First published in London, United Kingdom, 2019 by IntechOpen
IntechOpen is the global imprint of INTECHOPEN LIMITED, registered in England and Wales, registration number: 11086078, The Shard, 25th floor, 32 London Bridge Street
London, SE19SG - United Kingdom
Printed in Croatia

British Library Cataloguing-in-Publication Data
A catalogue record for this book is available from the British Library

Additional hard and PDF copies can be obtained from orders@intechopen.com

Selected Topics in Myasthenia Gravis
Edited by Isam Jaber Al-Zwaini and Ali AL-Mayahi
p. cm.
Print ISBN 978-1-83880-829-7
Online ISBN 978-1-83880-830-3
eBook (PDF) ISBN 978-1-83880-831-0

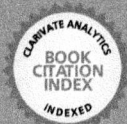

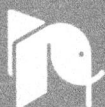

Meet the editors

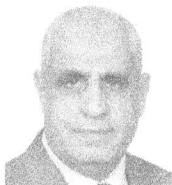

Prof. Isam Jaber Al-Zwaini was born on January 4, 1963, in Baghdad, Iraq. After graduating from Al-Mustansiryia College of Medicine in 1987, he worked as a house officer in different hospitals in Baghdad for 15 months, followed by military services for 3 years. He started his pediatric studies in 1991 and gained Fellowship of the Iraqi Commission for Medical Specializations in 1996. He worked as a lecturer in the Department of Pediatrics, Al-Anbar Medical College, from 1996 to 2001, where he was upgraded to assistant professor in 2008. In 2007, he gained associate membership of the Royal College of Paediatrics and Child Health, UK. He has been the head of the Pediatric Department in Al-Anbar and Al-Kindy Medical College for many years. He has published more than 30 scientific papers in different pediatric fields, and his special interests are pediatric hematology, neurology, and nutrition.

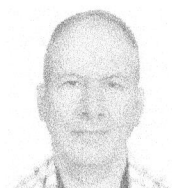

Assistant Professor Ali AL-Mayahi was born in Baghdad on September 11, 1968. He graduated from Al-Mustanisryia College of Medicine in 1992 and worked as a house officer for 2 years in Baghdad hospitals, before starting his pediatric specialty in 1994. He subsequently gained the degree of Fellowship of Iraqi Medical Specialization in 1999 and the Arab Board in Pediatrics in 2000. He then worked as a pediatric specialist at Kirkuk Welfare Hospital for Children and at Al-Elwyia Pediatric Teaching Hospital. Professor Al-Mayahi joined Al-Kindy College of Medicine, University of Baghdad, as a lecturer in 2006 and became an assistant professor in 2012. He was the head of the Pediatric Department at Al-Kindy College of Medicine from 2016 to 2018. His interests are neonatology, neurology, and hematology.

Contents

Preface

Myasthenia gravis (MG) is a rare potentially fatal chronic autoimmune disorder. Circulating autoantibodies directed against components of the neuromuscular junction of skeletal muscles, most commonly nicotinic acetylcholine receptor (nAChR) and associated protein in the postsynaptic membrane, block neuromuscular transmission resulting in muscle weakness. This muscle weakness typically worsens with continued activity, improves on rest, and is of variable severity ranging from mild ocular muscle weakness to severe generalized muscle weakness, involving the respiratory muscle with impending respiratory failure. The content of this short book is divided into three sections involving six chapters.

The first chapter is an Introductory chapter written by the editors, in which we trace the history of MG as a disease entity, which was reported in the Seventeenth century with the death of the Native American Chief Opechancanough in 1664. The chapter throws light on the etiology, epidemiology, pathophysiology, clinical presentations, diagnostic tests, and treatment of MG.

The second chapter written by Dr. Adel A. Kareem is dedicated to the myasthenic syndrome in children, which has special varieties whereby it may be inherited or acquired as an autoimmune disorder. Autoimmune MG is usually transient and is evident when a baby born to a myasthenic mother is floppy with a weak cry and suffers from ptosis and impaired respiration. Fortunately, most of these cases are transient and complete recovery will take place after a few weeks; however, these individuals need good supportive measures until recovery is ensured. On the other hand, classical autoimmune MG, which is known as juvenile MG, can occur at any childhood age group. An interesting occurrence in childhood myasthenia is congenital myasthenia syndrome, which is not uncommon. This nonimmunologic-mediated heterogeneous group has variable presentation, ranging from mild to severe weakness and respiratory failure.

Dr. Miljana Z. Jovandaric and Svetlana J. Milenkovic in the third chapter discuss the maternal and neonatal outcome of pregnancies with autoimmune MG. Transient neonatal MG is an uncommon type of MG affecting the newborns of mothers who suffer from the disorder or asymptomatic mothers having specific circulating autoantibodies. In most cases, the intensity of transient neonatal MG is not associated with the mothers' condition but rather with maternal antibody titers. The detection of the disease is generally possible several hours after birth. The symptoms of transient neonatal MG include hypotonia, feeding difficulties, weak cry, facial diplegia, and breathing difficulties in the affected newborns. These manifestations gradually disappear as maternally derived antibodies wane. Monitoring of these newborns is necessary for the first seven days after birth since during this period, transient neonatal myasthenic symptoms can be detected, especially on the second day.

The fourth chapter by Dr. Jiang Xu, Kaori Noridomi and Lin Chen reviews the structure-based approaches to antigen-specific therapy of MG. About 85% of cases of MG are caused by pathological autoimmune antibodies to muscle nAChRs. An attractive approach to treating MG is, therefore, blocking the binding of autoimmune antibodies to nAChRs, removing specific nAChR antibodies, or selectively inhibiting and eliminating nAChR-specific B cells. This chapter reviews high-resolution structural studies of muscle nAChR and its complexes with antibodies derived from experimental autoimmune MG. Based on these structural analyses, various strategies are used, including using small molecules to block the binding of MG autoimmune antibodies and engineered chimeric nAChR antigens to specifically target and eliminate B cells that produce nAChR-specific antibodies.

The fifth chapter by Prof. Valerii Voinov reviews the use of plasmapheresis in the treatment of MG. Treatment of MG is still a rather difficult task since there is no single tactic for using different drugs (corticosteroids, rituximab, and immunoglobulins), especially since they are associated with a number of side effects. They are not able to remove accumulating autoantibodies and immune complexes, the large size of which does not allow them to be excreted by the kidneys. Special problems of treatment arise when myasthenic crises develop with respiratory failure requiring artificial lung ventilation. Plasmapheresis can help with this, because it is possible to remove antibodies and other pathological metabolites. In addition, regular plasmapheresis is able not only to prevent exacerbations but also to reduce doses of maintenance therapy with reduced risk of their side effects.

The sixth chapter by Dr. Zeynep Özdemir and Mehmet Abdullah Alagöz gives an overview of anticholinesterases (AChEs). AChE and butyrylcholinesterase (BChE) are known serine hydrolase enzymes responsible for the hydrolysis of acetylcholine (ACh). Although the role of AChE in cholinergic transmission is well known, the role of BChE has not been elucidated sufficiently. The hydrolysis of ACh in synaptic healthy brain cells is mainly carried out by AChE. It is accepted that the contribution to the hydrolysis of BChE is very low, but both AChE and BChE are known to play an active role in neuronal development and cholinergic transmission. Pyridostigmine, distigmine, neostigmine, and ambenonium are the standard AChE drugs used in the symptomatic treatment of MG. All of these compounds may increase the response of the myasthenic muscle to recurrent nerve impulses, primarily by protecting the endogenous ACh.

Finally, I hope this short book with its interesting chapters will shed light on some of the fascinating aspects of MG. I would like to thank all authors who contributed with their chapters and for their patience and cooperation throughout the processing of the book. In addition, I would like to express my sincere appreciation and deep thanks and gratitude to the IntechOpen personnel, especially Ms. Anita Condic and Marijana Francetic who offered me great help throughout the processing of this book.

Isam Jaber Al-Zwaini, PhD
Professor
Department of Pediatrics, Al-Kindy Medical College,
University of Baghdad,
Baghdad, Iraq

Dr. Ali AL-Mayahi
AL-Kindy College of Medicine,
University of Baghdad,
Baghdad, Iraq

Section 1

Introduction

Chapter 1

Introductory Chapter: Myasthenia Gravis - An Overview

Isam Jaber AL-Zwaini and Ali AL-Mayahi

1. Introduction

The term myasthenia gravis (MG) is derived from the Greek terms my, asthenia, and gravis, which mean muscle, weakness, and severe, respectively. Myasthenia gravis is a rare potentially fatal chronic autoimmune disorder, in which circulating autoantibodies directed against components of the neuromuscular junction (NMJ) of skeletal muscles, most commonly nicotinic acetylcholine receptor (AChR) and associated protein in the postsynaptic membrane, will block neuromuscular transmission resulting in muscle weakness [1]. The muscle weakness is typically worsened with continued activity, improves on rest, and is of variable severity ranging from mild ocular muscle weakness to severe generalized muscle weakness involving the respiratory muscle with impending respiratory failure.

2. Historical perspective

The first reported case of MG could be traced to the Native American Chief Opechancanough, who died in 1664. "The excessive fatigue he encountered wrecked his constitution; his flesh became macerated; his sinews lost their tone and elasticity; and his eyelids were so heavy that he could not see unless they were lifted up by his attendants ...he was unable to walk; but his spirit rising above the ruins of his body directed from the litter on which he was carried by his Indians" [2, 3]. An English physician, Thomas Willis, in 1672 described a patient with a typical myasthenic fatigable weakness of limb and bulbar muscles [4]. The late 1800s certify the publishing first modern description of patients with myasthenia symptoms when Wilks in 1877 described bulbar and peripheral muscular weakness without any pathology of the central nervous system [5]. A great advance in understanding MG and its management were achieved in 1934 by Walker who found the symptoms of MG were similar to curare poisoning and was treated with a cholinesterase inhibitor, physostigmine. Walker showed that the symptoms of MG promptly improved by the administration of physostigmine [6]. In 1937, Blalock established the removal of thymus as a treatment for MG [4]. Simpson and Nastuck suggested the autoimmune etiology of MG in 1959–1960 [7, 8] depending on several observations. In the 1970s, prednisolone, azathioprine, and, later, plasma exchange were established as treatments for MG [2].

3. Epidemiology

The worldwide prevalence of MG is 100–200 per million population [9], affecting more than 700,000 people all over the world [10]. The prevalence rate

3

has increased since the 1950s due to improved diagnostic precision and decreased mortality rate. It occurs in both genders, in all ages from different ethnic groups with variable prevalence and annual incidence rate from one country to another. Female-to-male ratio for incidence is 3:2 in people below the age of 30 and 1:1.5 in people more than 50 years of age. Life-threatening MG crises occur approximately in 15–20% of patients, typically within the first 2 years of diagnosis [11]. Previously, MG crises were associated with 50–80% mortality rate. Currently, the overall inpatient mortality rate of MG is 2.2%, being higher in crises (4.47%). Older age and respiratory failure were the predictors for death in MG crises [12].

4. Etiology

Myasthenia gravis is an autoimmune disease mediated by organ-specific antibody. These antibodies are present at neuromuscular junction (NMJ) and directed against nicotinic acetylcholine receptor (AChR) on the postsynaptic muscle membrane in 80–90% of patients. In 3–7%, the autoantibodies are directed against another NMJ protein, muscle-specific tyrosine kinase (MuSK). Using cell-based assay may increase the rate of detection of autoantibodies in patients with negative result by standard binding and modulating technique [13]. Patients with negative antibodies against AChR and MuSK might show positive antibodies against low-density lipoprotein receptor-related protein (LRP4) [14]. Other types of antibodies might be detected in patients with MG like agrin antibodies and antibodies to collagen Q and cortactin. These antibodies are of debatable clinical importance [15]. The reason why some patients develop these autoantibodies remains unclear. Genetic predisposition linked to human leukocyte antigen complex, single nuclear polymorphism, association with thymic hyperplasia or thymoma and abnormalities in the number and function of regulatory T and B cells are probably playing a role in the etiology of MG [16–19]. Risk factors for developing MG include positive personal or family history of autoimmune disease like rheumatoid arthritis, HLA-B8, DR3, and women being less than 40 and men more than 60 years of age.

5. Pathophysiology

Normally, Ach is released in a discrete package from the motor nerve terminal at the neuromuscular junction. These Ach quanta diffuse across the synaptic cleft and bind to receptors on the folded muscle end plate membrane (**Figure 1**). Motor nerve stimulation will release many Ach quanta causing depolarization of muscle end plate membrane resulting in muscle contraction. In MG, Ach was released normally but its effect on the postsynaptic membrane reduced. The autoantibody against AChRs will result in the destruction of postsynaptic membrane and reduction in the number of available Ach receptors on the muscle end plate membrane (binding site for Ach), which in turn will lead to an inconsistent generation of muscular action potentials manifesting as muscle weakness (**Figures 2** and **3**). The process of destruction of the postsynaptic membrane is dependent on complement activation. In patients without antibodies against AChRs, a muscle-specific tyrosine kinase (MuSK), an agrin-dependent protein on muscle membrane, has been found to be the antigenic target. These

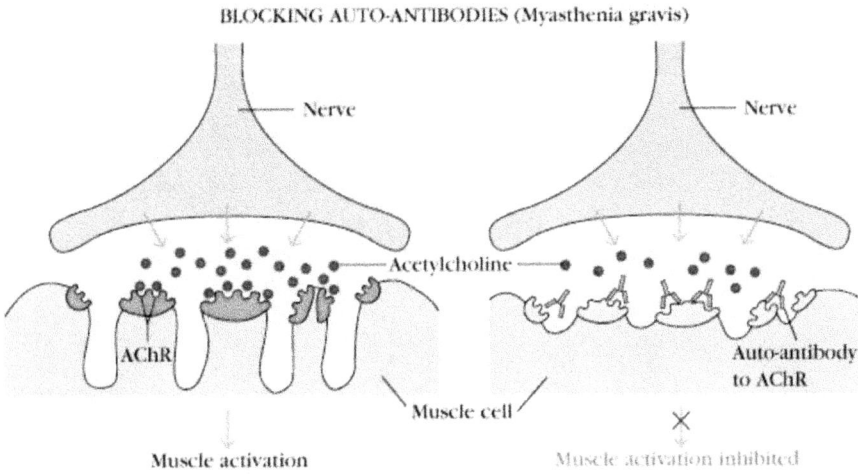

Figure 1.
Mechanism of muscle activation. Adopted from the free domain: http://pathologicallyspeaking.blogspot. com/2015/07/speech-therapy-treatment-for-myasthenia.htm.

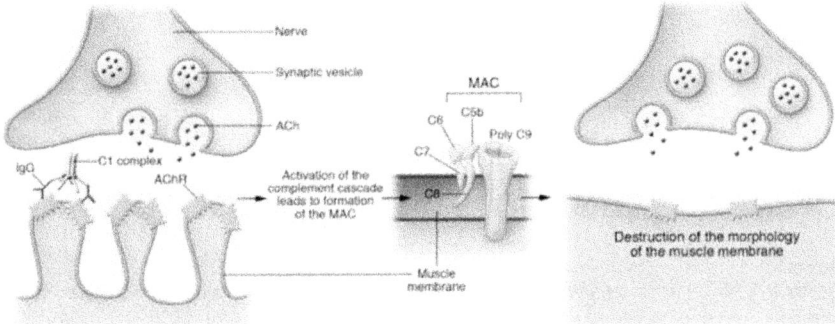

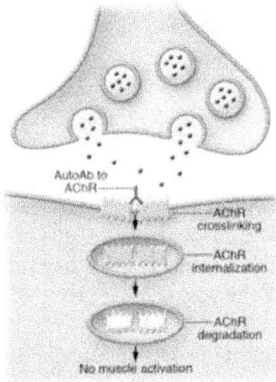

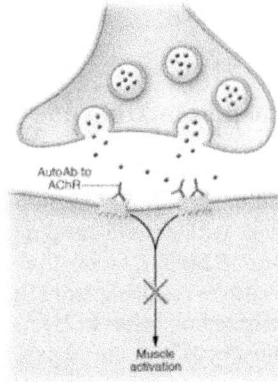

Figure 2.
Mechanisms of inhibition of neurotransmission by anti-AChR antibodies. Adopted from the free domain: https://www.jci.org/articles/view/29894/figure/2.

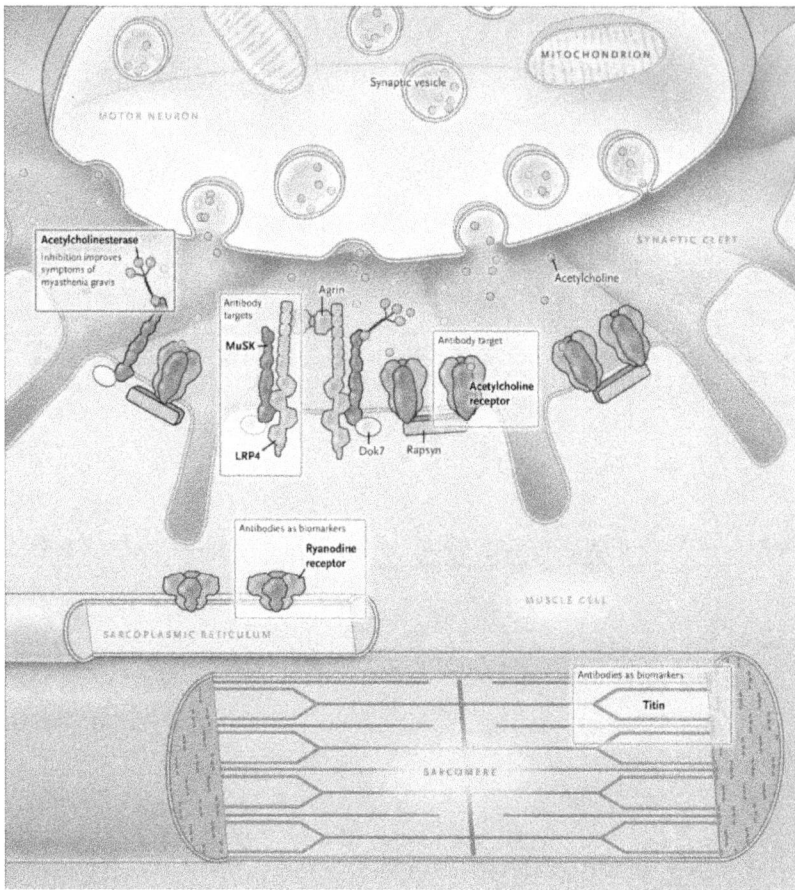

Figure 3.
Pathogenesis of MG. Adopted from the free domain: https://www.nejm.org/doi/full/10.1056/NEJMra1602678.

autoantibodies are T-cell dependent and there is interesting differential involvement of muscle groups, especially the extraocular muscles [20].

6. Clinical presentation

Fatigable weakness, involving specific susceptible groups of muscles, is the clinical hallmark of MG. This weakness usually fluctuates from hour to hour, day to day, worsens with activity, and improves on rest. The susceptible groups of muscles include ocular, bulbar, facial, limb muscle, axial muscle, and respiratory muscle. Clinical features resulting from the involvement of the susceptible group of muscle are summarized in **Table 1** [21].

The most common initial presenting feature of MG is ocular muscle involvement presenting as fluctuating ptosis and/or diplopia, with or without generalized weakness, in about 85% of cases [22]. The absence of ocular involvement makes the diagnosis difficult. In 50–60% of patients with isolated ocular involvement, progression to generalized weakness occurs within 2 years of the onset. The

Group of muscle	Clinical features
Ocular muscle	Fluctuating ptosis and/or diplopia
Bulbar muscle	Dysarthria, painless dysphagia, dysphonia, and masticatory weakness
Facial muscle	Facial weakness, inability to close eye firmly, drooling of saliva
Axial muscular	Flexion or extension of the neck
Limb muscle	Weakness involving the arms more than legs
Respiratory muscle	Labor breathing, orthopnea, dyspnea, and respiratory failure

Table 1.
Signs and symptoms of MG.

second most common presenting feature is bulbar muscle involvement manifesting as dysphagia, dysarthria, dysphonia, or difficulties in chewing, occurring in about 15% of cases [23]. A life-threatening respiratory muscle involvement, requiring immediate therapeutic action might occur on rare occasions. Patients with MG usually experience a variable course with intermittent worsening of symptoms precipitated by viral infection, surgery, warm weather, immunization, emotional stress, pregnancy, chronic diseases, or medications. Progression to maximum severity usually occurs with the first 2 years of onset and spontaneous long-term remission might occur in up to 10–20% of patients [22]. About 10–20% of infants born to mothers with symptomatic or asymptomatic MG present soon after birth with transient neonatal MG. It occurs as a result of transplacental passage of antibodies against NMJ receptors. The most common presenting features are hypotonia and poor feeding that resolve usually within the first months after birth [24].

7. Clinical classifications

Myasthenia gravis is classified clinically into five classes and several subclasses according to MG foundation of American clinical classification, see **Table 2** [25].

Class	Clinical description
Class 1	Any eye muscle weakness, possible ptosis, all other muscles' strength is normal
Class 2	Mild weakness of other muscles; may have eye muscle weakness of any severity
2a	Predominantly limb or axial muscles weakness or both
2b	Predominantly oropharyngeal or respiratory muscle weakness or both
Class 3	Moderate weakness of other muscles; may have eye muscle weakness of any severity
3a	Predominantly limb or axial muscle weakness or both
3b	Predominantly oropharyngeal or respiratory muscle weakness or both
Class 4	Severe weakness of other muscles; may have eye muscle weakness of any severity
4a	Predominantly limb or axial muscle weakness or both
4b	Predominantly oropharyngeal or respiratory muscle weakness or both; use of feeding tube without intubation
Class 5	Intubation needed to maintain airway

Table 2.
Clinical classification of MG.

8. Diagnosis

The diagnosis of MG might be difficult and easily missed, because of the rarity of the condition and hence unfamiliarity to physicians. Furthermore, fluctuations of muscle weakness may add to the perplexing presentation. Once MG is suspected, the following test can be requested:

8.1 Serological tests

Anti-AchR has about 100% specificity, 85% sensitivity in patients with generalized MG, and 50% sensitivity in pure ocular variety [26]. False positive results may occur in patients with thymoma without MG, small cell lung cancer, rheumatoid arthritis treated with penicillamine, and rarely in people over 70 years of age. Other serological tests include anti-MuSK antibody (positive in 50% of myasthenic patients with negative anti-AchR), anti-agrin antibody, anti-lipoprotein-related protein 4 (LRP4) antibody, antistriational antibody (present in all myasthenic patients with thymoma), and anti-cortactin antibody.

8.2 Neurophysiological studies

These studies are commonly used to detect defects in neuromuscular transmission in patients with MG. Repetitive nerve stimulation and single-fiber electromyography are the most commonly used tests. Repetitive nerve stimulation can detect 75 and <50% of generalized and ocular MG patients, respectively. On the other hand, single-fiber electromyography can detect defects in neuromuscular transmission in 95–99% of myasthenic patients and a negative result can exclude the diagnosis [27].

8.3 Radiological studies

Chest X ray, CT scan, and MRI might be recommended to evaluate patients with anterior mediastinal mass and suspected thymoma, and also to exclude brain and orbit mass lesion inducing cranial nerve palsies in ocular MG.

8.4 Pharmacological tests

In MG, the number of AChRs at the NMJ is low due to inhibition by the auto-antibody. The result is decrease in the number of interaction between Ach (release from motor nerve terminals) and its receptors on postsynaptic muscle membrane of NMJ. The Ach is metabolized by Ach esterase (AChE) enzyme. Therefore, inhibition of this enzyme will increase the Ach concentration at the NMJ and hence improve the chance of interaction between the Ach and its receptors. Edrophonium test is based on the clinical improvement of muscle weakness in myasthenic patients after intravenous administration of short-acting Ach esterase inhibitor, Edrophonium (Tensilon). Double blinding of both the patient and the examiner increases the validity of the test [28].

8.5 Ice pack test

This debatable test uses the fact that cooling might improve neuromuscular transmission. It is mainly used by ophthalmologists to assess improvement in ptosis and diplopia in myasthenic patients [29].

9. Treatment

The severity of symptoms in patients with MG will determine the strategy of the treatment using the many therapeutic options available. According to MG foundation of American clinical classification (**Table 2**), MG can be divided into three categories: mild (classes 1 and 2), moderate (class 3), and severe (classes 4 and 5). The available therapeutic options include:

9.1 Pharmacologic therapy

The cornerstone for the treatment of MG is the administration of reversible cholinesterase (AChE) inhibitor, pyridostigmine, which is more effective in patients with generalized and ocular MG and less effective in patients with positive anti-MuSK antibody. In those patients with poor response to pyridostigmine, steroid and immunosuppressive agents should be considered [30–32].

9.2 Immunosuppressive agent

All types of MG respond to corticosteroid (prednisone and prednisolone) in terms of improvement of muscle strength. Furthermore, corticosteroid may prevent progression of the disorder from ocular to generalized MG [30, 33]. Patients who do not respond to corticosteroid or who cannot tolerate it are candidates for immunosuppressive agents using azathioprine (they are first-line agents and can be used with corticosteroid), cyclosporine, methotrexate, mycophenolate mofetil, or tacrolimus [32]. Recently, promising results are shown by two monoclonal antibodies, rituximab and eculizumab. The use of rituximab in refractory MG may show clinical improvement and reduction for the need of corticosteroid and therapeutic plasma exchange [34].

9.3 Therapeutic plasma exchange (TPE)

It is the procedure by which the patient's plasma is removed and replaced by fresh plasma or albumin. This will lead to the removal of autoantibody against AChRs, leading to short-term improvement of NMJ transmission and hence muscular strength. It is useful as an acute treatment in patients with severe generalized MG, refractory MG, myasthenia crises, and as maintenance therapy in patients with juvenile MG [35].

9.4 Intravenous immunoglobulin (IVIG)

The mechanism of action of IVIG is complex and may involve inhibition of cytokines and complement deposition, competition with autoantibodies, interference with binding of Fc receptor on macrophages and immunoglobulin receptor on B cells, and interference with antigen recognition by sensitized T cells [36]. It is used as an acute treatment in patients with severe generalized MG and MuSK-MG, as a maintenance therapy in patients with refractory and juvenile MG, and in myasthenia crises [1].

9.5 Thymectomy

Myasthenic patients commonly have thymic abnormalities. Patients with generalized MG have thymic hyperplasia in 85% and thymoma in 10–15% of cases. Those patients are usually anti-AChR antibody positive. Thymectomy is indicated for all patients with thymoma and for patients aged 10–55 years who have generalized MG but without thymoma. In fact, thymectomy is proposed as first – line therapy in most patients with generalized MG. Thymectomy not indicated in patients with antibodies to MuSK, LRP4, or agrin antibodies because the thymic pathology is different from the more common type of MG characterized by seropositivity to AChR, and also it is not indicated in patients with ocular MG during the first 2 years after diagnosis because the possibility of spontaneous remission [2].

10. Prognosis

With the recent advances in the management of MG in both supportive intensive care and specific therapeutic options, most patients enjoy normal or near normal life span. The mortality rate is about 3–4% and the risk factors for death include a short history of a progressive disease, age more than 40 years, and thymoma. Morbidity in MG results from intermittent muscle weakness, which may result in aspiration pneumonia, difficult breathing, and even respiratory failure requiring ventilator assistance and in possible side effects of medications used in the treatment.

Author details

Isam Jaber AL-Zwaini[1*] and Ali AL-Mayahi[2]

1 Department of Pediatrics, AL-Kindy Medical College, University of Baghdad, Iraq

2 AL-Kindy College of Medicine, University of Baghdad, Baghdad, Iraq

*Address all correspondence to: isamjaber@kmc.uobaghdad.edu.iq

IntechOpen

References

[1] Kernich CA. Patient and family fact sheet. Myasthenia gravis: Maximizing function. The Neurologist. 2008;**14**(1):75-76

[2] Conti-Fine BM, Milani M, Kaminski HJ. Myasthenia gravis: Past, | present, and future. The Journal of Clinical Investigation. 2006;**116**(11):2843-2854

[3] Marsteller HB. The first American case of myasthenia gravis. Archives of Neurology. 1988;**45**:185-187

[4] Pascuzzi RM. The history of myasthenia gravis. Neurologic Clinics. 1994;**12**:231-242

[5] Wilks S. On cerebritis, hysteria and bulbar paralysis, as illustrative of arrest of function of the cerebrospinal centres. Guy's Hospital Reports. 1877;**22**:7-55

[6] Walker MB. Case showing the effect of prostigmin on myasthenia gravis. Proceedings of the Royal Society of Medicine. 1935;**28**:759-761

[7] Nastuk WL, Strauss AJ, Osserman KE. Search for a neuromuscular blocking agent in the blood of patients with myasthenia gravis. The American Journal of Medicine. 1959;**26**:394-409

[8] Simpson JA. Myasthenia gravis, a new hypothesis. Scottish Medical Journal. 1960;**5**:419-436

[9] Phillips LH. The epidemiology of myasthenia gravis. Seminars in Neurology. 2004;**24**:17-20

[10] Sanders DB, Wolfe GI, Benatar M, Evoli A, Gilhus NE, Illa I, et al. International consensus guidance for management of myasthenia gravis. Neurology. 2016;**87**(4):419-425

[11] Liu CJ, Chang YS, Teng CJ, et al. Risk of extrathymic cancer in patients with myasthenia gravis in Taiwan: A nationwide population-based study. European Journal of Neurology. 2012;**19**(5):746-751

[12] Alshekhlee A, Miles JD, Katirji B, Preston DC, Kaminski HJ. Incidence and mortality rates of myasthenia gravis and myasthenic crisis in US hospitals. Neurology. 2009;**72**(18):1548-1554. DOI: 10.1212/WNL.0b013e3181a41211

[13] Meriggioli MN, Sanders DB. Muscle autoantibodies in myasthenia gravis: Beyond diagnosis? Expert Review of Clinical Immunology. 2012;**8**(5):427-438

[14] Higuchi O, Hamuro J, Motomura M, et al. Autoantibodies to low-density lipoprotein receptor-related protein 4 in myasthenia gravis. Annals of Neurology. 2011;**69**(2):418-422

[15] Cossins J, Belaya K, Zoltowska K, et al. The search for new antigenic targets in myasthenia gravis. Annals of the New York Academy of Sciences. 2012;**1275**:123-128

[16] Giraud M, Vandiedonck C, Garchon HJ. Genetic factors in autoimmune myasthenia gravis. Annals of the New York Academy of Sciences. 2008;**1132**:180-192

[17] Renton AE, Pliner HA, Provenzano C, et al. A genome-wide association study of myasthenia gravis. JAMA Neurology. 2015;**72**(4):396-404

[18] Hohlfeld R, Wekerle H. The role of the thymus in myasthenia gravis. Advances in Neuroimmunology. 1994;**4**(4):373-386

[19] Vander Heiden JA, Stathopoulos P, Zhou JQ, et al. Dysregulation of B cell repertoire formation in myasthenia gravis patients revealed through deep sequencing. Journal of Immunology. 2017;**198**(4):1460-1473

[20] Hughes BW, Moro De Casillas ML, Kaminski HJ. Pathophysiology of myasthenia gravis. Seminars in Neurology. 2004;**24**:21-30

[21] Meriggioli MN, Sanders DB. Autoimmune myasthenia gravis: Emerging clinical and biological heterogeneity. Lancet Neurology. 2009;**8**(5):475-490

[22] Grob D, Brunner N, Namba T, Pagala M. Lifetime course of myasthenia gravis. Muscle & Nerve. 2008;**37**:141-149

[23] Grob D. Course and management of myasthenia gravis. Journal of the American Medical Association. 1953;**153**:529-532

[24] Hassoun M, El Turjuman U, Chokr I, Fakhoury H. Myasthenia gravis in the neonate. NeoReviews. 2010;**11**(4):e200-e205. DOI: 10.1542/neo.11-4 e200

[25] Jaretzki A 3rd, Barohn RJ, Ernstoff RM, et al. Myasthenia gravis: Recommendations for clinical research standards. Task force of the medical scientific advisory board of the myasthenia Gravis foundation of America. The Annals of Thoracic Surgery. 2000;**70**(1):327-334

[26] Padua L, Stalberg E, LoMonaco M, Evoli A, Batocchi A, Tonali P. SFEMG in ocular myasthenia gravis diagnosis. Clinical Neurophysiology. 2000;**111**(7):1203-1207

[27] Katirji B, Kaminski HJ. Electrodiagnostic approach to the patient with suspected neuromuscular junction disorder. Neurologic Clinics. 2002;**20**:557-586, viii

[28] Phillips LH 2nd, Melnick PA. Diagnosis of myasthenia gravis in the 1990s. Seminars in Neurology. 1990;**10**(1):62-69

[29] Benatar M. A systematic review of diagnostic studies in myasthenia gravis. Neuromuscular Disorders. 2006;**16**(7):459-467

[30] Skeie GO, Apostolski S, Evoli A, et al. Guidelines for treatment of autoimmune neuromuscular transmission disorders. European Journal of Neurology. 2010;**17**(7):893-902

[31] Gilhus NE, Owe JF, Hoff JM, Romi F, Skeie GO, Aarli JA. Myasthenia gravis: A review of available treatment approaches. Autoimmune Diseases. 2011;**2011**:847393

[32] Saperstein DS, Barohn RJ. Management of myasthenia gravis. Seminars in Neurology. 2004;**24**(1):41-48

[33] Benatar M, Kaminski H. Medical and surgical treatment for ocular myasthenia. Cochrane Database of Systematic Reviews. 2012;**12**:CD005081

[34] Nowak RJ, Dicapua DB, Zebardast N, Goldstein JM. Response of patients with refractory myasthenia gravis to rituximab: A retrospective study. Therapeutic Advances in Neurological Disorders. 2011;**4**(5):259-266

[35] Kumar R, Birinder SP, Gupta S, Singh G, Kaur A. Therapeutic plasma exchange in the treatment of myasthenia gravis. Indian Journal of Critical Care Medicine. 2015;**19**(1):9-13

[36] Eng H, Lefvert AK, Mellstedt H, Osterborg A. Human monoclonal immunoglobulins that bind the human acetylcholine receptor. European Journal of Immunology. 1987;**17**:1867-1869

Section 2

Pediatric Myasthenia Gravis

Chapter 2

Myasthenic Syndrome in Children

Adel A. Kareem

Abstract

The myasthenic syndrome in children can be inherited or of acquired autoimmune origin. In the autoimmune syndrome, babies born to a myasthenic mother are floppy at birth with weak cry, ptosis, and impaired respiration. Fortunately, most of these cases are transient and complete recovery will take place after few weeks; however, good supportive measures are needed until recovery. On the other hand, the classical autoimmune myasthenia gravis (MG), which is known as juvenile myasthenia gravis, can occur in children of any age group. It is commonly divided into prepubertal and postpubertal, the latter usually follows adult criteria, is more common in females, generalized, and most of them are seropositive for neuromuscular antibodies. In contrast, in acquired myasthenia gravis that occurs in prepubertal children, there is no sex predilection and patients are less likely seropositive, and ocular myasthenia more likely to occur than postpubertal. An interesting group of childhood myasthenic syndromes is the congenital myasthenic syndrome; this is an uncommon, nonimmune-mediated heterogeneous syndrome with variable presentation, ranging from mild symptoms with little weakness to severe ones that may cause extreme weakness and respiratory failure. Congenital myasthenic syndrome is classified into presynaptic, synaptic, and postsynaptic, and each of them has subtypes, with the postsynaptic syndrome representing the most common type. Many patients with congenital myasthenic syndrome are misdiagnosed with seronegative acquired myasthenia or congenital myopathy; however, advances in disease investigation are showing promise in early and precise diagnosis.

Keywords: myasthenia gravis, congenital myasthenic syndrome, neonatal myasthenia

1. Introduction

Myasthenia gravis in children generally is not uncommon disease, either it is genetic type known as congenital myasthenia syndrome (CMS) that involve structural defect of neuromuscular junction [1]. It is significant that is included in the differential diagnosis of seronegative myasthenia gravis (MG), congenital myopathy, peripheral neuropathy, and childhood and adolescent motor neuron diseases.

The prevalence rates of acquired autoimmune myasthenia gravis on the other hand have been increasing in the last two decades, with approximately 20 cases per 100,000 in the US population. In this syndrome, autoantibodies act against the neuromuscular junction (NMJ) [2].

Furthermore, there is another type of syndrome called transient neonatal myasthenia in which there is a passive transfer of autoantibodies from a mother with myasthenia gravis (MG).

The primary manifestation is weakness typically with diurnal fluctuation; nevertheless, variant or atypical presentations must also be considered and appropriately recognized.

MG is suspected from clinical and neurological examinations, particularly fatigue test. Moreover, investigation tools like electromyography (EMG) with repetitive stimulation tests and special instances may need the use of single fibers.

In general, advances in intensive care, therapy, and the use of immunomodulatory agents are improving the quality of life of patients with MG.

2. Congenital myasthenic syndrome

Congenital myasthenic syndrome (CMS) is a genetic disease, inherited as autosomal recessive, nonimmunologic neuromuscular disorder, with a prevalence of about 1/200,000. Its onset occurs usually at infancy, although sometimes its presentation can be delayed to young adulthood. Weakness along with fatigue is major presentation of CMS, and repetitive nerve stimulations have revealed decremental response in CMS patients in the absence of antibodies against muscle or neuromuscular junction [1, 3].

3. Classification of congenital myasthenic syndrome

Usually classified according to the defective site of the neuromuscular junction, it is often divided into presynaptic, synaptic, and postsynaptic disorders (**Table 1**) [4].

Presynaptic CMS: the prototype is CMS with episodic apnea, which is genetically determined as mutations in the enzyme choline acetyltransferase (ChAT) [5, 6]. Moreover, other presynaptic disorders have been detected that have a paucity of synaptic vesicles release with features resembling the autoimmune Lambert-Eaton myasthenic syndrome [7].

Synaptic CMS: solely related to acetylcholinesterase (AChE) deficiency in which there are mutations in COLQ, it is the second most common cause of CMS (about 15%), coding for the collagen-like tail of the AChE molecule [8, 9].

Congenital myasthenic syndrome (CMS)	Presynaptic defects (5%)	Synaptic defect (basal lamina) (15%)	Postsynaptic defects (80%)
	Choline acetyltransferase deficiency	Endplate acetylcholinesterase deficiency	Reduced AChR expression
	Paucity of synaptic vesicles		AChR mutations
	Congenital Lambert-Eaton-like syndrome		Rapsyn mutations
	Other unclassified presynaptic defects		DOK-7 mutations
			AChR kinetic abnormality
			Slow-channel syndrome
			fast-channel syndrome
			Sodium-channel mutations

AChR, acetylcholine receptor.

Table 1.
Classification of congenital myasthenic syndromes [7, 15].

Postsynaptic CMS: in which a variety of genes have been detected to encode the AChR subunits, resulting in defects in AChR function or AChR subunit deficiencies like congenital myasthenia associated with Dok-7 deficiency and sodium-channel myasthenia or their combinations. In general, AChR mutation represents the majority of CMSs, about 75–85% [1, 3, 10, 11]. Furthermore, mutations in the genes for rapsyn and muscle-specific receptor tyrosine kinase (MuSK) reduced AChR expression and are considered an important cause of postsynaptic CMS [12].

4. Clinical presentations of congenital myasthenic syndromes

There are no constant clinical features for the diagnosis of CMS, and it is based on the age of presentation and type of neuromuscular defect; however, a nonspecific clue of the syndrome might be evident prenatally, which is reduced fetal movement. Neonates and infants with CMS experience generalized weakness, delayed motor milestone, and hypotonia with an evidence of wasted muscle bulk over time along with an evidence of exertional weakness and fluctuation of weakness, which gets worse with intercurrent infection. Various skeletal deformities are usually observed like high-arched palate, dysmorphic facial features, arthrogryposis, and scoliosis [4].

4.1 Presynaptic CMS

4.1.1 Congenital myasthenic syndrome with episodic apnea

Congenital myasthenic syndrome with episodic apnea represents an exemplary standard of presynaptic CMS, an autosomal recessive disorder with mutations in the gene encoding choline acetyltransferase (ChAT) [4].

The baby is described at birth as floppy with irregular breathing and difficulty in feeding. Examinations show ptosis with mild extraocular muscle weakness; however, the baby experiences recurrent apneic episodes, which is considered as a hallmark of this disorder. Nonetheless, apneic episodes may occur with other types of CMSs also; so, CMS with episodic apnea may be a misnomer. Prolonged apnea may lead to brain damage due to hypoxia. The apnea is usually precipitated by stressful conditions like fever, infection, and exertion. Therefore, CMS must be considered in differential diagnosis in families with history of sudden infant death. The apnea in this type of CMS decreases with advancing of age and will respond to anticholinesterase medication such as pyridostigmine prophylaxis [4].

Although EMG remains the initial diagnostic procedure in suspected cases, it often shows normal repetitive nerve stimulation at low rate (3 Hz), and single-fiber EMG (SFEMG) is usually normal. But a decremental response is found at prolonged exertion or high-rate (10 Hz) repetitive nerve simulation [4].

4.2 Synaptic CMS

4.2.1 Congenital acetylcholinesterase (AChE) deficiency

Congenital acetylcholinesterase (AChE) deficiency is an autosomal recessive disorder that presents with hypotonia and weakness that is often significant and involves the face. There are also delayed motor millstones, feeding difficulties, and, sometimes, skeletal deformities like scoliosis. Moreover, the patient may have peculiar finding such as pupillary hyporeflexia and progressive myopathy. Unfortunately, the patient does not respond or may get worse with anticholinesterase or other medication that is used for other types of CMS; however, some cases respond to ephedrine [13].

EMG displays usual features of neuromuscular disorders with decremental compound muscle action potential (CMAP) with repeated nerve stimulation in addition to jitter with single-fiber electromyography (SFEMG). On the other hand, there is an interesting EMG finding, which occurs in AChE deficiency in addition to the slow-channel syndrome, and this is repeated CMAP in response to single nerve stimulation.

The pathophysiology behind that is prolonged exposure of acetylcholine (Ach) to its receptor due to defect in its destruction by absence or defect in AChE, in consequence there is muscle membrane depolarizing block [14, 15].

4.3 Postsynaptic CMS

The postsynaptic CMS is considered the most common type of CMS and is caused by gene mutations that encode AChR subunits. In consequence, there is a defect in ion-channel gating and or a decrease in number of receptors resulting in slow-channel, fast-channel, or AChR deficiency syndrome; in addition, the mutation may be in the rapsyn, MuSK, or Dok-7, resulting in neuromuscular junction disorders [11, 16].

4.3.1 AChR deficiency

AChR deficiency is inherited as autosomal recessive with mutation in genes that encode AChR subunits in the postsynaptic neuromuscular junction. Clinically, the patient presents early in infancy with variable severity; the child experiences motor developmental delay, ptosis, limitation of extraocular movement, and impaired feeding. However, it is not progressive, and weakness improves to some extent when the child becomes older.

EMG displays typical myasthenic syndrome features that include decremental CMAPs at low-rate (3 Hz) stimulations and increasing jitters with block in single-fiber EMG [17].

4.3.2 Kinetic abnormality of the AChR

The functional character and kinetic properties of AChR may be impaired as a result of mutation in AChR deficiency gene, particularly when AChR is not significantly reduced. Slow-channel and fast-channel CMSs represent the main kinetic abnormalities of the AChR.

4.3.2.1 Slow-channel congenital myasthenic syndrome (SCCMS)

SCCMS is considered the most common type of CMS [1]. The primary pathogenesis is increased duration of channel opening resulting from kinetic impairment of AChR. In consequence, there is slowing of the rate of channel closure with an increase in the rate of channel opening; moreover, sometime increase receptor-AChE affinity resulting in depolarizing neuromuscular block and weakness with exertion. It is an autosomal dominant inheritance with variable penetrance and expression in most cases; however, autosomal recessive inheritance has also been reported [18, 19]. Its presentation had variable severity and variable age of onset from early infancy, which could be delayed to teenage. Clinical manifestation is characterized by muscular weakness and wasting involving neck and scapular and extensor muscles of finger. Ptosis and extraocular muscle involvement mild or spared. The circumstances have been different from other types of CMS, this type usually progressive although its slowly, furthermore respiratory muscle and other muscles particularly upper limb, intrinsic and fingers extensor muscles in addition to bulbar muscles are regularly involved [19].

EMG must be done to the involved muscle for sensitive results; and usually, it shows decremental CMAP in low-rate (3 Hz) stimulations. Interestingly, like endplate AChE deficiency, single-nerve stimulation usually but not always shows unique repetitive CMAP response [20].

SCCMS must be considered in the differential diagnosis of congenital muscular dystrophy, congenital myopathy, autoimmune-type MG, and metabolic and mitochondrial myopathy.

Patients with SCCMS like AChE deficiency get worse with the use of cholinesterase inhibitors due to enhanced desensitization of receptors via prolonged endplate current, which gives clue to differentiate this syndrome from autoimmune MG; however, if the patient does not receive treatment, the symptoms get worse in consequent years. Quinidine and fluoxetine are considered the medication of choice, their action on decrease opening of AChR channel [21, 22]. The dose of quinidine is 200 mg; when given twice or three times per day, it leads to improvement in short- and long-term weakness and even improved nerve conductivity as detected by EMG follow-up. In practice, fluoxetine with a dose of 80–160 mg per day is preferable as it has less side effects with same effectiveness as quinidine [15].

4.3.2.2 Fast-channel congenital myasthenic syndrome

Fast-channel congenital myasthenic syndrome is an autosomal recessive inheritance and has common features with AChR deficiency syndromes; however, it is more severe. The pathophysiology disparity to SCCMS in which Ach., when bound to Ach receptor, the time of channel opening is short, in consequence the activation become short resulting in decrease transmission of signals [11, 23, 24]. Clinically, it is like other CMSs presenting with delayed motor milestones, ptosis, limitation of extraocular movement with difficulties in feeding and chewing, and also fatigue and generalized weakness triggered by exertion [25]. Nonetheless, mild cases may be missed clinically and even via EMG procedures and erroneously diagnosed as congenital myopathy. In contrast, the severe cases experience respiratory distress, facial involvement or even arthrogryposis multiplex features [1]. Of note, fast-channel CMS must be considered in differential diagnosis of patients with seronegative myasthenic syndrome.

EMG findings show typical symptoms of postsynaptic neuromuscular disorders that include decremental CMAPs at repetitive low-rate simulations (3 Hz), increased jitter with block in single-fiber EMG, and no observation of repetitive CMAPs.

Fortunately, the patient benefits from the use of cholinesterase inhibitors and 3,4-diaminopyridine or both [26] and if left without treatment may experience slowly progressive disease or remain stationary.

4.3.3 Mutations affecting acetylcholine receptor (AChR) clustering and synaptic structure

To achieve effective synaptic transmission, there must be functional and structural integrity of all involved neuromuscular postsynaptic parts [27].

4.3.3.1 AChR deficiency due to receptor-associated protein of the synapse (RAPSN) mutations

AChR deficiency due to receptor-associated protein of the synapse (RAPSN) mutations may occur at any age; nevertheless, neonates are the most commonly affected and might need nasogastric tubes for feeding and mechanical ventilation due to severe hypotonia and significant bulbar involvement. Sometimes, the baby is born with arthrogryposis multiplex, but the condition improves with advancing age with less probability of apnea. It is sometimes misdiagnosed as seronegative acquired autoimmune myasthenia gravis. Ankle dorsiflexion weakness is considered a characteristic feature of this syndrome and might give hint for the diagnosis [28].

EMG; as other myasthenic syndrome show decremental CMAP and jitter in single fiber. Nevertheless, sometimes, there is difficulty in detection of these typical features in EMG.

Fortunately, those patients respond to anticholinesterase agents and may get additional improvement from 3,4-diaminopyridine [28].

4.3.3.2 Congenital myasthenic syndrome with proximal weakness due to mutations in DOK7

This syndrome is sometimes called limb girdle CMS as proximal muscle weakness is more than that of the distal one [29]. Although the patient initially attained millstones on time, but the patient might have ptosis since early infancy and could be progressive on the other hand in childhood age experience progressive weakness with predominant proximal muscle weakness and may lead to nonambulation state. Fifty percent of patients display tongue atrophy and ptosis which might be progressive, but often still no ophthalmoplegia and the fluctuation of symptoms are predominant nevertheless a lot of patients misdiagnosed as myopathies [30, 31].

4.3.3.3 Mutations in CHRNG neuromuscular transmission

Mutations in CHRNG neuromuscular transmission is caused by prenatal inherited myasthenia, which in consequence might result in fetal developmental abnormalities [32].

Escobar's syndrome (multiple pterygium syndrome) is the most well-known type of CMS attributed to CHRNG mutation. It is inherited as autosomal recessive with cranial deformities including ptosis, low-set ear, high-arched palate, receded chin, and orthopedic deformities including arthrogryposis multiplex and cervical pterygia; in addition, many of them die in the uterus [33].

4.3.3.4 MuSK mutations postsynaptic CMS

The mutation impairs postsynaptic voltage-gated sodium channel (SCN4A) and might cause severe respiratory distress with fluctuation of disease severity. Unfortunately, patients do not respond to anticholinesterases but might respond well to combined therapy with diaminopyridine [34, 35].

5. Childhood autoimmune myasthenia gravis

Generally, there is no significant difference in myasthenia gravis between patients younger than 18 years and adults in terms of pathophysiology, clinical presentation, and diagnosis [36, 37]. CMS must be considered in seronegative MG, but low incidence of seropositive cases in acquired MG makes the diagnosis challengeable. There is no female predominance with higher rate of spontaneous remission in prepubertal children. On other hand, there is evidence of higher prevalence of ocular MG in prepubertal children [38].

Although the treatment line is the same as that of adults, there is concern of stunted growth with steroid treatment, as well as the drawback of accumulative effect of immunosuppressive drugs [39, 40]. Thymectomy is usually postponed as there is a possibility of spontaneous remission to happen and attempt to avoid such invasive procedure. Therefore, the treatment should be individualized, and generally, the treatment is often less aggressive, particularly in the prepubertal age group.

Although respiratory failure might occur in some cases, the general prognosis is often satisfactory.

6. Neonatal myasthenia caused by maternal MG

Maternal MG can cause transient neonatal myasthenia in about 20% of cases, the pathophysiology behind is AChR autoantibodies cross the placenta from the mother to the fetus. The neonate may have born with severe weakness to mother with mild MG and the invers is true, therefore, the severity of disease in neonate is not related to mother MG. Moreover, it is not related to the duration of maternal MG and can occur even in those with seronegative MG [41–44]. Nevertheless, the effect may have decreased with proper maternal treatment, while subsequent pregnancy may cause more affected neonates [45–47].

The condition is usually transient, and it presents clinically soon after birth with generalized weakness, difficulty in sucking and swallowing, weak cry, respiratory distress, which may get worse with inability to clear pharynx that may cause airway obstruction and cyanosis, in addition to ptosis and strabismus, but it is less common in older children.

The diagnosis is suspected by history of maternal MG, detection of AChR antibody in the infant and mother, and EMG—older children show decremental response with low rate of repetitive stimulation but not for high rates as decremental response occurs in high-rate stimulations in normal neonates. Furthermore, responding to cholinesterase inhibitors make diagnosis most likely [48].

Treatment involves cholinesterase inhibitors, in addition to supportive measures. Plasma exchange may be needed for severe, life-threatening conditions.

The prognosis fortunately is good as the syndrome is transient and improvement is complete in most infants with the duration of recovery ranging from 1 week to 8 weeks without recurrence, which is most probably related to the clearance of causative autoantibodies. However, about 10% of patients may die because of inadequate respiratory support and delayed or improper treatment [49].

7. Conclusion

Myasthenia syndrome in children not uncommon but the unique in children is the inherited congenital myasthenia syndrome which is not follow autoimmune and no antibodies determined. Therefore, a precise diagnosis is important for treatment. The challenge is to differentiate this syndrome from seronegative acquired myasthenia gravis and one may need, in addition to conventional investigation, specialized microelectrode analysis of neuromuscular transmission with or without genetic test.

Author details

Adel A. Kareem
Welfare Teaching Hospital, Baghdad, Iraq

*Address all correspondence to: adelkareemlh@gmail.com

IntechOpen

References

[1] Engel AG, Sine SM. Current understanding of congenital myasthenic syndromes. Current Opinion in Pharmacology. 2005;**5**(3):308-321

[2] Phillips LH II. The epidemiology of myasthenia gravis. Annals of the New York Academy of Sciences. 2003;**998**:407-412

[3] Engel AG, Ohno K, Sine SM. Sleuthing molecular targets for neurological diseases at the neuromuscular junction. Nature Reviews Neuroscience. 2003;**4**:339-352

[4] Beeson D, Hantai D, Lochmuller H, Engel AG. 126th International Workshop: Congenital Myasthenic Syndromes, 24-26 September 2004, Naaden, the Netheralnds. Neuromuscular Disorders. 2005;**15**:498-512

[5] Ohno K, Tsujino A, Brengman JM, et al. Choline acetyltransferase mutations cause myasthenic syndrome associated with episodic apnea in humans. Proceedings of the National Academy of Sciences of the United States of America. 2001;**98**:2017-2022

[6] Maselli RA, Chen D, Mo D, Bowe C, Fenton G, Wollmann RL. Choline acetyltransferase mutations in myasthenic syndrome due to deficient acetylcholine resynthesis. Muscle & Nerve. 2003;**27**:180-187

[7] Milone M, Fukuda T, Shen XM, Tsujino A, Brengman J, Engel AG. Novel congenital myasthenic syndromes associated with defects in quantal release. Neurology. 2006;**66**:1223-1229

[8] Donger C, Krejci E, Serradell AP, et al. Mutation in the human acetylcholinesterase-associated collagen gene, COLQ, is responsible for congenital myasthenic syndrome with endplate acetylcholinesterase deficiency (Type 1c). American Journal of Human Genetics. 1998;**63**:967-975

[9] Ohno K, Brengman J, Tsujino A, Engel AG. Human endplate acetylcholinesterase deficiency caused by mutations in the collagen-like tail subunit (ColQ) of the asymmetric enzyme. Proceedings of the National Academy of Sciences of the United States of America. 1998;**95**:9654-9659

[10] Sine SM, Ohno K, Bouzat C, et al. Mutation of the acetylcholine receptor alpha subunit causes a slow-channel myasthenic syndrome by enhancing agonist binding affinity. Neuron. 1995;**15**:229-239

[11] Ohno K, Wang HL, Milone M, et al. Congenital myasthenic syndrome caused by decreased agonist binding affinity due to a mutation in the acetylcholine receptor epsilon subunit. Neuron. 1996;**17**:157-170

[12] Muller JS, Baumeister SK, Schara U, et al. CHRND mutation causes a congenital myasthenic syndrome by impairing co-clustering of the acetylcholine receptor with rapsyn. Brain. 2006;**129**(pt 10):2784-2793

[13] Bestue-Cardiel M, Saenz de Cabezon-Alvarez A, et al. Congenital endplate acetylcholinesterase deficiency responsive to ephedrine. Neurology. 2005;**65**:144-146

[14] Hutchinson DO, Walls TJ, Nakano S, et al. Congenital endplate acetylcholinesterase deficiency. Brain. 1993;**116**(pt 3):633-653

[15] Michel Harper C. Congenital myasthenic syndrome. CONTINUUM: Lifelong Learning in Neurology. 2009;**15**(1):63-82

[16] Ohno K, Hutchinson DO, Milone M, et al. Congenital myasthenic syndrome

caused by prolonged acetylcholine receptorchannel openingsdue to a mutation in the M2 domainof the epsilon subunit. Proceedings of the National Academy of Sciences of the United States of America. 1995;**92**:758-762

[17] Vincent A, Cull-Candy SG, Newsom-Davis J, Trautmann A, Molenaar PC, Polak RL. Congenital myasthenia: Endplate acetylcholine receptors and electrophysiology in five cases. Muscle & Nerve. 1981;**4**:306-318

[18] Engel AG, Ohno K, Milone M, et al. New mutations in acetylcholine receptor subunit genes reveal heterogeneity in the slow-channel congenital myasthenic syndrome. Human Molecular Genetics. 1996;**5**(9):1217-1227

[19] Croxen R, Hatton C, Shelley C, et al. Recessive inheritance and variable penetrance of slow-channel congenital myasthenic syndromes. Neurology. 2002;**59**:162-168

[20] Quiram PA, Ohno K, Milone M, et al. Mutation causing congenital myasthenia reveals acetylcholine receptor beta/delta subunit interaction essential for assembly. The Journal of Clinical Investigation. 1999;**104**:1403-1410

[21] Harper CM, Engel AG. Quinidine sulfate therapy for the slow-channel congenital myasthenic syndrome. Annals of Neurology. 1998;**43**(4):480-484

[22] Harper CM, Fukodome T, Engel AG. Treatment of slow-channel congenital myasthenic syndrome with fluoxetine. Neurology. 2003;**60**(10):1710-1713

[23] Brownlow S, Webster R, Croxen R, et al. Acetylcholine receptor delta subunit mutations underlie a fast-channel myasthenic syndrome and arthrogryposis multiplex congenita. The Journal of Clinical Investigation. 2001;**108**(1):125-130

[24] Shen XM, Ohno K, Fukudome T, et al. Congenital myasthenic syndrome caused by low-expressor fast-channel AChR delta subunit mutation. Neurology. 2002;**59**(12):1881-1888

[25] Wang HL, Milone M, Ohno K, et al. Acetylcholine receptor M3 domain: Stereochemical and volume contributions to channel gating. Nature Neuroscience. 1999;**2**:226-233

[26] Engel G. The therapy of congenital myasthenic syndromes. Neurotherapeutics. 2007;**4**(2):252-257

[27] Sanes JR, Lichtman JW. Induction, assembly, maturation and maintenance of a postsynaptic apparatus. Nature Reviews Neuroscience. 2001;**2**:791-805

[28] Burke G, Cossins J, Maxwell S, et al. Rapsyn mutations in hereditary myasthenia; distinct early- and late-onset phenotypes. Neurology. 2003;**61**:826-828

[29] McQuillen MP. Familial limb-girdle myasthenia. Brain. 1966;**89**:121-132

[30] Palace J, Lashley D, Newsom-Davis J, et al. Clinical features of the DOK7 neuromuscular junction synaptopathy. Brain. 2007;**130**:1507-1515

[31] Muller JS, Herczegfalvi A, Vilchez JJ, et al. Phenotypical spectrum of DOK7 mutations in congenital myasthenic syndromes. Brain. 2007;**130**:1497-1506

[32] Mishina M, Takai T, Imoto K, et al. Molecular distinction between fetal and adult forms of muscle acetylcholine receptor. Nature. 1986;**321**:406-411

[33] Escobar V, Bixler D, Gleiser S, Weaver DD, Gibbs T. Multiple pterygium syndrome. American Journal of Diseases of Children. 1978;**132**:609-611

[34] Chevessier F, Faraut B, Ravel-Chapuis A, et al. MuSK, a new target

for mutations causing congenital myasthenic syndrome. Human Molecular Genetics. 2004;**13**:3229-3240

[35] Tsujino A, Maertens C, Ohno K, et al. Myasthenic syndrome caused by mutation of the SCN4A sodium channel. Proceedings of the National Academy of Sciences of the United States of America. 2003;**100**:7377-7382

[36] Parr JR, Jayawant S. Childhood myasthenia: Clinical subtypes and practical management. Developmental Medicine and Child Neurology. 2007;**49**(8):629-635

[37] Andrews PI. Autoimmune myasthenia gravis in childhood. Seminars in Neurology. 2004;**24**(1): 101-110

[38] Batocchi AP, Evoli A, Palmisani MT, LoMonaco M, Bartoccioni M, Tonali P. Early onsetmyasthenia gravis: Clinical characteristics and response to therapy. European Journal of Pediatrics. 1990;**150**:66-68

[39] Della Marina A, Trippe H, Lutz S, Schara U. Juvenile myasthenia gravis: Recommendations for diagnostic approaches and treatment. Neuropediatrics. 2014;**45**(2):75-83

[40] Matthews HJ, Thambundit A, Allen BR. Anti-MuSK-positive myasthenic crisis in a 7-year-old female. Case Reports in Emergency Medicine. 2017;**2017**:8762302

[41] Eymard B, Vernet-der Garabedian B, Berrih-Aknin S, Pannier C, Bach JF, Morel E. Antiacetylcholine receptor antibodies in neonatal myasthenia gravis: Heterogeneity and pathogenic significance. Journal of Autoimmunity. 1991;**4**:185-195

[42] Namba T, Brown SB, Grob D. Neonatal myasthenia gravis: Report of two cases and review of the literature. Pediatrics. 1970;**45**:488-504

[43] Papazian O. Transient neonatal myasthenia gravis. Journal of Child Neurology. 1992;**7**:135-141

[44] Melber D. Maternal-fetal transmission of myasthenia gravis with acetylcholine-receptor antibody. The New England Journal of Medicine. 1988;**318**:996

[45] Vernet-der Garabedian B, Lacokova M, Eymard B, et al. Association of neonatal myasthenia gravis with antibodies against the fetal acetylcholine receptor. The Journal of Clinical Investigation. 1994;**94**:555-559

[46] Hoff JM, Daltveit AK, Gilhus NE. Myasthenia gravis in pregnancy and birth: Identifying risk factors, optimizing care. European Journal of Neurology. 2007;**14**:38-43

[47] Gardnerova M, Eymard B, Morel E, et al. The fetal/adult acetylcholine receptor antibody ratio in mothers with myasthenia gravis as a marker for transfer of the disease to the newborn. Neurology. 1997;**48**:50-54

[48] Weis GA, McQuillen MP. Transient neonatal myasthenia gravis: Clinical and electromyographic studies. Archives of Neurology. 1970;**22**:556-565

[49] Djelmis J, Sostarko M, Mayer D, Ivanisevic M. Myasthenia gravis in pregnancy: Report on 69 cases. European Journal of Obstetrics, Gynecology, and Reproductive Biology. 2002;**104**:21-25

Chapter 3

Maternal and Neonatal Outcome of Pregnancies with Autoimmune Myasthenia Gravis

Miljana Z. Jovandaric and Svetlana J. Milenkovic

Abstract

Myasthenia gravis (MG) is an autoimmune neuromuscular disease manifested by the weakness and fatigue in skeletal muscles of the face and extremities. Transient neonatal myasthenia gravis is an uncommon type of MG affecting the newborns with mothers who suffer from the disorder or specific circulating autoantibodies. In most cases, the intensity of transient neonatal MG is not associated with the mothers' condition but rather with maternal antibody titers. The symptoms of transient neonatal MG are hypotonia, feeding difficulties, weak cry, facial diplegia, and breathing difficulties in the affected newborns. The disease is connected to the passive transplacental transfer of anti-acetylcholine receptor antibodies (anti-AChR) or antimuscle-specific tyrosine kinase antibodies (anti-MuSK) from the affected mother to the infant. The postsynaptic neuromuscular junction is damaged by the circulation of autoimmune antibodies, and the antibodies directed against fetal AChR are responsible for the form of fetal onset. Monitoring of these newborns is necessary in the first 7 days upon birth, since during this period of life, TNM symptoms can be detected, especially on the second day. In pregnancy period, myasthenia gravis symptoms may vary and they frequently worsen, sometimes leading to premature delivery.

Keywords: neonates, pregnancy, autoimmune myasthenia gravis

1. Introduction

Myasthenia gravis (MG) is a chronic progressive disease which is manifested in weakness and tiredness of skeletal muscles as most typical symptoms. Neuromuscular transmission defects are responsible for MG onset [1].

The expression "myasthenia gravis" is of Latin origin, where "myasthenia" means "muscle weakness" and "gravis" means "serious" or "heavy." The first report on MG was recorded in 1672 by Thomas Willis (1621–1675), a doctor from England whose main area of research was the nervous system [2].

Although patients suffering from myasthenia gravis do not experience any changes in the nervous and muscular systems, this disease causes a disorder in the transmission of the impulse from the nerve to the muscle, resulting in muscle weakness which is a typical symptom of neurological diseases. One of the most recognizable signals of this disease is the fluctuating weakness in the eyes, bulbar, limbs, and respiratory muscles [3, 4].

MG can be defined as a relatively rare autoimmune disorder, affecting approximately 2 out of every 100,000 people, and can develop at any age. In patients affected by MG, antibodies are formed against acetylcholine nicotinic postsynaptic receptors at the neuromuscular junction of skeletal muscles which leads to progressive skeletal muscle weakness [5]. Myasthenia gravis usually affects female population at the age ranging from 18 to 25, whereas male population is affected by this disease later in life, at the age ranging from 60 to 80 [6].

Depending on the affected skeletal muscle groups, myasthenia gravis is categorized into several classes:

- Class I: Only ocular muscles are weakened with possible weakness of eye closure, while other muscles remain unaffected.

- Class II: Mild weakness of any muscle group is possible as well as ocular muscle weakness of any degree.

- Class IIa: Most commonly causes weakness in limb and axial muscles; occurrence of oropharyngeal muscle weakness is also possible.

- Class IIb: Usually affects either oropharyngeal or respiratory muscles, but it can affect both muscle groups as well; limb and/or axial muscles can also be involved.

- Class III: Mild weakness of any muscle group is possible as well as ocular muscle weakness of any degree.

- Class IIIa: Most commonly causes weakness in limb and axial muscles; occurrence of oropharyngeal muscle weakness is also possible.

- Class IIIb: Usually affects either oropharyngeal or respiratory muscles, but it can affect both muscle groups as well; limb and/or axial muscles can also be involved.

- Class IV: Severe weakness of any muscle group is possible as well as ocular muscle weakness of any degree.

- Class IVa: Most commonly causes weakness in limb and axial muscles; occurrence of oropharyngeal muscle weakness is also possible

- Class IVb: Usually affects either oropharyngeal or respiratory muscles, but it can affect both muscle groups as well; limb and/or axial muscles can also be involved; application of a feeding tube without intubation.

- Class V: Characterized by the necessity of intubation, with or without mechanical ventilation, with the exception of cases of its application in routine postoperative management [7].

2. Myasthenia gravis during pregnancy

Myasthenia gravis can affect the courses of pregnancy and delivery, and it also presents a risk factor for the neonates [8]. On the other hand, pregnancy can intensify the symptoms of myasthenia which can lead to complications during pregnancy and require a modified treatment. Attention should be paid to ensure an optimal treatment and drug safety before conception. Myasthenia gravis can be transferred to neonates. However, neonatal myasthenia gravis is a treatable and transient disease [9]. MG is relatively frequent in the reproductive period of 1/10,000 to 1/50,000 [10].

The clinical course of MG can be altered unpredictably, and in various ways by pregnancy and the previous pregnancy, experiences are not a reliable source of information on the possible clinical course of subsequent pregnancies [11, 12].

In pregnancy, respiratory function of the lungs is compromised for two reasons. Hypoventilation caused by respiratory muscle weakness, on the one side, and diaphragm elevation caused by fetus growth on the other side lead to the reduction of the lung capacity [13].

MG symptoms can be worsened by puerperal respiratory and urinary tract infections; in order to avoid further complications, a prompt diagnosis and adequate antibiotic treatment of these infections is necessary during pregnancy [14].

It should be taken into consideration that the selected groups of antibiotics—for example, fluoroquinolones (such as moxifloxacin and ciprofloxacin), macrolides (such as azithromycin and erythromycin), and aminoglycosides (such as streptomycin and gentamicin)—can aggravate muscle weakness caused by MG; therefore, these types of antibiotics should be avoided [15].

During pregnancy therapy administration has to be based on individual conditions and symptoms regarding the groups of muscles affected by MG in each patient, bearing in mind the possible side effects and consequences on the fetus [16].

For the symptomatic treatment of myasthenia gravis in the period of pregnancy, acetylcholinesterase inhibitors can be chosen. In most cases of MG during pregnancy, immunosuppressant corticosteroids are effective and hence should be selected in accordance with the symptoms in specific cases of MG [17].

Occurrence of premature membrane rupture and preterm delivery were also reported in cases when patients were treated with high doses of corticosteroids. There are records on temporary increase of MG symptom severity triggered by the introduction of corticosteroid therapy. Although the introduction of immunosuppressive drugs should be avoided before and during pregnancy, therapy reduction or discontinuation bears the risk of triggering a myasthenic crisis or exacerbation in pregnant myasthenic women. In order to control the teratogenic risk to the fetus, immunosuppressive drug dosages have to be carefully balanced and individualized [18].

On the other hand, recent reports suggest that azathioprine (AZA) therapy has shown to be successful in treatments of MG during pregnancy and breastfeeding periods. Even though AZA is absorbed through the placenta, its negative effects on the fetus are relatively minor since the fetal liver is immature and lacks the enzyme responsible for the conversion of AZA into its active metabolites. Cyclosporine A treatment is not considered to be harmful during the period of pregnancy and breastfeeding, but it can also trigger prematurity, spontaneous abortions, and insufficient birth weight at birth. Another drug, mycophenolate mofetil (MMF), is thought to be teratogenic, causing a clinical syndrome which includes hypoplastic nails, shortened fifth fingers, oral cleft, microtia, diaphragmatic hernia, and micrognathia [19].

MG rarely affects the first stage of delivery, mostly because in this stage smooth muscles are involved. However, in the second stage, the mother can experience fatigue due to the involvement the voluntary striated muscles [20].

In this stage of delivery, mothers frequently feel exhausted, which may involve myasthenic crisis; therefore, the obstetrician needs to be ready for an assisted vaginal delivery if required (e.g., performing vacuum extraction or using forceps) [21].

Since MG patients are particularly sensitive to a number of anesthetics, an anesthesiologist should be consulted at the beginning of the pregnancy. Both in vaginal and in surgical deliveries, epidural anesthesia not exceeding the tenth thoracic vertebra level is advisable in order to ensure an adequate analgesia. While amide-type local anesthetic agents (such as lidocaine, mepivacaine, and bupivacaine) have no impact on myasthenia, ester-type drugs (e.g., benzocaine, tetracaine, and procaine) are not the drug of choice because of the risk of aggravation of the existing myasthenia. Nonsteroidal anti-inflammatory medications (e.g., ketorolac tromethamine) and paracetamol (acetaminophen) may be included to ease postpartum or postoperative pain, while narcotic analgesic agents that can contribute to respiratory depression are to be avoided [22].

Although anti-acetylcholine therapy can be used safely by nursing mothers suffering from MG, it may exacerbate symptoms of transient *neonatal myasthenia gravis* (TNMG), since anti-acetylcholine receptor antibodies (AChR-Ab) are contained in breast milk [23, 24].

Glucocorticoids and AZA are also not contraindicated in myasthenic mothers, but a liver function test must be performed, and complete blood count must be monitored in the newborns breastfed by myasthenic mothers. However, in breast-feeding mothers with MG, mycophenolate mofetil is contraindicated [23].

Taking care of the newborn can be particularly strenuous for myasthenic mothers due to the lack of sleep at night and constant daily caring for the infant. These extreme efforts may worsen the clinical symptoms of MG. In cases where immunosuppressive therapy has to be initiated or restarted after giving birth, contraceptive counseling is strongly recommended. A carefully chosen contraceptive has to be prescribed a minimum of 1 month prior to the initiation of immunosuppressive therapy, and it should not be discontinued 6 months prior to a new pregnancy. A cyclic withdrawal of oral contraceptives has been reported to initiate worsening of MG symptoms. In such cases, continuous hormonal contraception or an intrauterine device is more preferable [25].

3. Newborns by myasthenic mothers

Neonatal MG is typically triggered by an autoactivation of the immune system. The causative factor is not known, but the disorder may have a genetic defect, leading to congenital MG, or placental transmission of maternal antibodies, resulting in transient neonatal MG. TNM is a temporary condition caused by transplacental circulation of mothers' antibodies. It develops in 10–20% cases of infants with myasthenic mothers, due to transplacental circulation of mothers' antibodies [26, 27].

In these infants general muscle weakness is noticeable together with deficient suck, lethargy, and breathing difficulty until the fourth day upon birth. These symptoms are considered to be the consequence of transplacental transfer of antibodies. However, this causative effect is somewhat unclear, since a close correlation has neither been found between the severity of MG in mothers and existence of neonatal myasthenia nor between neonatal myasthenia gravis and maternal anti-AChR antibody titers. The correlation might be explained by the protective role of alpha-fetoprotein in neonatal myasthenia gravis, as alpha-fetoprotein has been proven to inhibit the binding of myasthenia gravis antibody to its receptor [28, 29].

Premature delivery occurs in approximately 35% of cases of mothers. The most common fetal abnormalities are pulmonary hypoplasia and arthrogryposis. Death from malformations attributable to myasthenia gravis has also been reported [30].

Although TNMG can potentially be a life-threatening condition, it can have excellent prognosis if it is timely identified and properly treated [31].

Transient neonatal myasthenia gravis (TNMG) is a rare form of MG which affects the infants whose mothers have the disorder or specific circulating autoantibodies [32].

There are cases in which the mother is asymptomatic. The level of severity is not necessarily connected with the mother's condition but rather with maternal antibody titers. The onset is typically shown immediately after birth. The recognizable symptoms in infants affected by TNMG are hypotonia, feeding difficulties, weak cry, facial diplegia, and respiratory distress in the affected neonates. Most commonly, these symptoms recede gradually with the decrease in maternally derived antibodies. The risk of this disorder continues for the subsequent births. The exact risk factors for the condition are yet to be identified. If treated promptly, the symptoms resolve within 2 months upon birth [33, 34].

TNMG is connected to the passive transplacental transfer of anti-acetylcholine receptor antibodies (anti-AChR) or anti-muscle-specific tyrosine kinase antibodies (anti-MuSK) from the affected mother to the infant. The postsynaptic neuromuscular junction is damaged by the circulation of autoimmune antibodies, and the antibodies directed against fetal AChR are responsible for the form of fetal onset [35].

The pathogenic role of acetylcholine receptor (AChR) antibodies has not been precisely determined. Despite the fact that passive-transfer acetylcholine receptor (AChR) antibodies are identified in most of these neonates, only a small percentage of infants develop the symptoms. A biological marker for prenatal detection of this group of neonates has not been identified yet, but recent reports suggest that HLA typing can be used successfully for this purpose. Final diagnosis can be given when the therapy of acetylcholinesterase agents temporarily improves the neuromuscular transmission disorder. Serum AChR antibody titers behave in the same way as the maternal pattern.

Anticholinesterase agents and supportive management before breastfeeding are required in approximately 80% of cases. The symptoms disappear spontaneously in most cases [27, 36, 37].

4. Conclusion

Newborns of mothers with MG manifest clinical features of TNM relative to the phase of the mothers' disease and transplacental transfer of antibodies to acetylcholine receptors throughout the placenta. These newborns need to be monitored until their seventh day of life, as TNM symptoms can be visible from birth to 7 days of life, though most commonly on the second day of life. The clinical course of myasthenia gravis during pregnancy is variable, with a significant proportion of patients experiencing worsening of clinical symptoms and premature delivery.

Conflict of interest

No potential conflict of interest was reported by the authors.

Funding

None.

Author details

Miljana Z. Jovandaric* and Svetlana J. Milenkovic
Department of Neonatology, Clinic for Gynecology and Obstetrics, Clinical Center
of Serbia, Belgrade, Serbia

*Address all correspondence to: rrebecca080@gmail.com

IntechOpen

References

[1] Bourque PR, Breiner A. Myasthenia gravis. CMAJ. 2018;**190**:E1141

[2] Drachman DB. Myasthenia gravis. The New England Journal of Medicine. 1994;**330**:1797-1810

[3] Grob D, Brunner N, Namba T, Pagala M. Lifetime course of myasthenia gravis. Muscle & Nerve. 2008;**37**:141-149

[4] Khanna S, Liao K, Kaminski HJ, Tomsak RL, Joshi A, Leigh RJ. Revitalized ocular myasthenia: Insights from pseudo-intercellular ophthalmoplegia. Journal of Neurology. 2007;**254**:1569-1574

[5] Barber C. Diagnosis and management of myasthenia gravis. Nursing Standard. 2017;**31**:42-47

[6] Niks EH, Verrips A, Semmekrot BA, et al. A transient neonatal myasthenic syndrome with anti-musk antibodies. Neurology. 2008;**70**:1215-1216

[7] Jaretzki A III, Jaretzki A 3rd, Barohn RJ, Ernstoff RM, Kaminski HJ, Keesey JC, et al. Myasthenia gravis: Recommendations for clinical research standards. Task force of the medical scientific advisory board of the myasthenia gravis foundation of America. Neurology. 2000;**55**:16-23

[8] Pijnenborg JM, Hansen EC, Brölmann HA, Oei SG, Andriessen P, Dellemijn PL. A severe case of myasthenia gravis during pregnancy. Gynecologic and Obstetric Investigation. 2000;**50**:142-143

[9] Hamel J, Ciafaloni E. An update: Myasthenia gravis and pregnancy. Neurologic Clinics. 2018;**36**:355-365

[10] Roth CK, Dent S, McDevitt K. Myasthenia gravis in pregnancy. Nursing for Women's Health. 2015;**19**:248-252

[11] Wenninger S, Schoser B. Myasthenia gravis: Current status of antibody diagnostics and aspects on refractory myasthenia gravis. Fortschritte der Neurologie-Psychiatrie. 2018;**86**:551-558

[12] Djelmis J, Sostarko M, Mayer D, Ivanisevic M. Myasthenia gravis in pregnancy: Report on 69 cases. European Journal of Obstetrics & Gynecology and Reproductive Biology. 2002;**104**:21-25

[13] Plauché WC. Myasthenia gravis in mothers and their newborns. Clinical Obstetrics and Gynecology. 1991;**34**:82-99

[14] Van Bambeke F, Harms JM, Van Laethem Y, Tulkens PM. Ketolides: Pharmacological profile and rational positioning in the treatment of respiratory tract infections. Expert Opinion on Pharmacotherapy. 2008;**9**:267-283

[15] Elsais A, Popperud TH, Melien Ø, Kerty E. Drugs that may trigger or exacerbate myasthenia gravis. Tidsskrift for den Norske Lægeforening. 2013;**133**:296-299

[16] Ciafaloni E, Massey JM. The management of myasthenia gravis in pregnancy. Seminars in Neurology. 2004;**24**:95-100

[17] Stafford IP, Dildy GA. Myasthenia gravis and pregnancy. Clinical Obstetrics and Gynecology. 2005;**48**:48-56

[18] Imai T, Utsugisawa K, Murai H, Tsuda E, Nagane Y, Suzuki Y, et al. Oral corticosteroid dosing regimen and long-term prognosis in generalized myasthenia gravis: A multicenter cross-sectional study in Japan. Journal of Neurology, Neurosurgery, and Psychiatry. 2018;**89**:513-517

[19] Norwood F, Dhanjal M, Hill M, James N, Jungbluth H, Kyle P, et al. Myasthenia in pregnancy: Best practice guidelines from a U.K. multispecialty working group. Journal of Neurology, Neurosurgery, and Psychiatry. 2014;**85**:538-543

[20] Ducci RD, Lorenzoni PJ, Kay CS, Werneck LC, Scola RH. Clinical follow-up of pregnancy in myasthenia gravis patients. Neuromuscular Disorders. 2017;**27**:352-357

[21] Massey JM, De Jesus-Acosta C. Pregnancy and myasthenia gravis. Continuum. 2014;**20**:11527

[22] Hassan A, Yasawy ZM. Myasthaenia gravis: Clinical management issues before, during and after pregnancy. Sultan Qaboos University Medical Journal. 2017;**17**:e259-e267

[23] Varner M. Myasthenia gravis and pregnancy. Clinical Obstetrics and Gynecology. 2013;**56**:372-381

[24] Papazian O. Transient neonatal myasthenia gravis. Journal of Child Neurology. 1992;**7**:135-141

[25] Khadilkar SV, Sahni AO, Patil SG. Myasthenia gravis. The Journal of the Association of Physicians of India. 2004;**52**:897-904

[26] Cheng I, Lin CH, Lin MI, Lee JS, Chiu HC, Mu SC. Outcome of myasthenia gravis mothers and their infants. Acta Paediatrica Taiwanica. 2007;**48**:141-145

[27] Oger J, Frykman H. An update on laboratory diagnosis in myasthenia gravis. Clinica Chimica Acta. 2015;**449**:43-48

[28] Saint-Faust M, Perelman S, Dupont D, Velin P, Chatel M. Transient neonatal myasthenia gravis revealing a myasthenia gravis and a systemic lupus erythematosus in the mother: Case report and review of the literature. American Journal of Perinatology. 2010;**27**:107-110

[29] Hoff JM, Daltveit AK, Gilhus NE. Myasthenia gravis in pregnancy and birth: Identifying risk factors, optimising care. European Journal of Neurology. 2007;**14**:38-43

[30] Maddison P. Myasthenia gravis and pregnancy: Pressing time for best practice guidelines. Journal of Neurology, Neurosurgery, and Psychiatry. 2014;**85**:477

[31] Qi QW, Wang D, Liu JT, Bian XM. Management of pregnancy with myasthenia gravis: 7 cases report. Zhonghua Fu Chan Ke Za Zhi. 2012;**47**:241-244

[32] Gajda A, Szabó H, Gergev G, Karcagi V, Szabó N, Endreffy E, et al. Congenital myasthenic syndromes and transient myasthenia gravis. Ideggyógyászati Szemle. 2013;**66**:200-203

[33] Edmundson C, Guidon AC. Neuromuscular disorders in pregnancy. Seminars in Neurology. 2017;**37**:643-652

[34] Eymard B, Morel E, Dulac O, Moutard-Codou ML, Jeannot E, Harpey JP, et al. Myasthenia and pregnancy: A clinical and immunologic study of 42 cases (21 neonatal myasthenia cases). Revue Neurologique. 1989;**145**:696-701

[35] Eymard B. Antibodies in myasthenia gravis. Revista de Neurologia. 2009;**165**:137-143

[36] D'Amico A, Bertini E, Bianco F, et al. Fetal acetylcholine receptor inactivation syndrome and maternal myasthenia gravis: A case report. Neuromuscular Disorders. 2012;**22**:546-548

[37] Ramirez C, de Seze J, Delrieu O,
Stojkovic T, Delalande S, Fourrier F,
et al. Myasthenia gravis and pregnancy:
Clinical course and management
of delivery and the postpartum
phase. Revista de Neurologia.
2006;**162**:330-338

Section 3

Myasthenia Gravis - Therapeutic Aspects

Chapter 4

Structure-Based Approaches to Antigen-Specific Therapy of Myasthenia Gravis

Jiang Xu, Kaori Noridomi and Lin Chen

Abstract

A majority of Myasthenia Gravis (MG) cases (~85%) are caused by pathological autoimmune antibodies to muscle nicotinic acetylcholine receptors (nAChRs). An attractive approach to treating MG is therefore blocking the binding of autoimmune antibodies to nAChR, or removing specifically nAChR antibodies, or selectively inhibiting and eliminating nAChR-specific B cells. This chapter will review high-resolution structural studies of muscle nAChR and its complexes with antibodies derived from experimental autoimmune Myasthenia Gravis (EAMG). Based on these structural analyses, various strategies, including using small molecules to block the binding of MG autoimmune antibodies, and engineered chimeric nAChR antigen to specifically target and eliminate B cells that produce nAChR-specific antibodies, will be discussed.

Keywords: crystal structure, nicotinic acetylcholine receptor, antigen-specific therapy, Myasthenia Gravis, autoimmune antibodies, chimeric nAChR antigen, nAChR-specific B cells

1. Introduction

Myasthenia Gravis (MG) is an autoimmune disease that afflicts a significant human population. MG patients suffer from a variable degree of skeletal muscle weakness. The symptoms range from mere lack of muscle strength to life-threatening respiratory failure. MG is a chronic disease that can last many years and negatively impact the quality of living and life expectancy of afflicted individuals. Although MG rate is reported to be 7–20 out 100,000 [1] and the diagnosed MG cases are increasing, probably due to increased awareness of this debilitating disease, the aging population and other intrinsic and extrinsic factors that disturb the human immune system [1].

The majority of MG cases (~85%) are caused by pathological autoantibodies to muscle nicotinic acetylcholine receptors (nAChRs), a ligand-gated ion channel that mediates rapid signal communication between spinal motor neurons and the muscle cells. Autoantibodies against other neuromuscular junction (NMJ) proteins, including muscle-specific kinase (MuSK) and lipoprotein-related protein 4 (LRP4), can also cause muscle weakness in a small fraction of patient [2, 3]. The heterogeneous nature of MG autoantibody presents a challenge to both diagnosis and treatment of the disease.

Current treatment regimens for MG include anticholinesterase inhibitors, thymectomy, immunosuppressants, plasmapheresis, or intravenous immunoglobulins [4].

Most MG patients respond favorably to these treatment options to achieve effective symptom relief, and in some cases even clinical remission. Cholinesterase inhibiting drugs can temporarily enhance neuromuscular transmission by delaying the breakdown of acetylcholine (ACh) to compensate for the loss of NMJ nAChRs, but this treatment option only works in a fraction of patients and does not alter the autoimmune response. The more broadly used nonspecific immunosuppressive drugs work by inhibiting lymphocyte activation and proliferation but have little effect on long-lived plasma cells that are terminally differentiated and continue producing pathogenic antibodies [5, 6]. This may explain why treatment with nonspecific immunosuppressive drugs takes long time to show clinical improvement.

There are two major limitations in the current MG treatment. First, up to 10% of MG patients do not tolerate or are resistant to the available treatments [7]. Second, all immunosuppressant drugs, which are often used in the long-term control of chronic MG, inevitably carry the serious risks of infection and cancer. As such continued efforts have been put into searching for better MG treatment, as evident by the long list of clinical trials (ClinicalTrials.gov) testing well known immunosuppressive drugs such as methotrexate and azathioprine, as well as new biologics agents such as the anti-CD20 monoclonal antibody rituximab (which depletes B cells) and the anticomplement C5 monoclonal antibody eculizumab.

An ideal therapeutic approach to MG would be to inhibit the pathogenic autoimmune response to nAChR specifically without disrupting other functions of the immune system. Because nAChR is a dominant autoantigen in MG, it has served as the primary target for a wide range of studies attempting to develop antigen-specific therapy to induce immune tolerance to nAChR [8–14]. While some of these approaches showed promising results in animal model of experimental autoimmune MG (EAMG), translation to human MG treatment is uncertain. Furthermore, introducing an autoantigen like nAChR or its derivative peptides risks to inadvertently enhance the pathogenic autoimmune response.

Here, we will first review structural and molecular features of nAChR and its complexes with autoantibodies. Based on insights derived from structural studies, we will discuss several strategies to specifically inhibit the binding of pathological autoantibodies to nAChR or specifically eliminate nAChR-specific B cells.

2. Structural study of nAChR

As the first isolated neurotransmitter receptor and ion channel, nicotinic acetylcholine receptors (nAChRs) have been the focus of extensive studies to understand the basic mechanisms of neuronal signaling. These receptors are also being targeted for drug development against a variety of diseases, including addiction, depression, attention-deficit/hyperactivity disorder (ADHD), schizophrenia, Alzheimer's disease, pain and inflammation [15]. nAChRs have been analyzed by a variety of biochemical, biophysical and electrophysiological experiments [16]. Tremendous efforts have been put into pursuing the atomic structure of nAChR. Electron microscopic analyses of nAChR from *Torpedo marmorata* by Unwin and colleagues have led to a 4 Å resolution model of the intact channel [17, 18], providing one of the most comprehensive structural model for nAChR. The structural details, however, are limited by the relatively low resolution. In this regard, the high-resolution structure of the acetylcholine binding protein (AChBP) published by Sixma and colleagues in 2001 was a major breakthrough [19]. AChBP shares ~24% sequence identity with nAChRs and has the same pentameric assembly. Its structures in different bound states have provided detailed information on the binding of a variety of agonists and antagonists [20]. But AChBP does not function as an ion channel and may lack necessary structural features required for transmitting the ligand-binding signal across the protein body [21, 22]. The crystal structures of several prokaryotic homologues of nAChR have also been determined from different species and in different states [23–25]. These structures together with detailed biochemical and biophysical characterization have provided a great deal of insight into the fundamental mechanisms of ligand-dependent channel gating (reviewed in Corringer et al [26]). More recently, the structure of the anionic glutamate receptor (GluCl) from *C. elegans* [27], and human $\alpha4\beta2$ neuronal nicotinic receptor have also been determined [28]. However, direct structural information of mammalian muscle nAChRs at high resolution will be needed for further dissecting the mechanisms of neuromuscular junction signal transmission and for drug development against MG [29].

3. High-resolution structural analysis enabled by stabilizing nAChR mutants

Although large quantities of nAChR were available from *Torpedo* electric ray organ, crystallization was not successful, probably due to the heterogeneity of the protein samples prepared from the natural source. Heterologous expression in bacterial results in insoluble protein is due to the lack of proper post translation modifications such as glycosylation. Yeast *Pichia pastoris* has been a favorable expression system for overexpressing nAChR because of its mammalian-like glycosylation system. However, the expressed nAChR protein or extracellular domain (ECD) is often unstable, leading to aggregation and low yield [30, 31]. We have employed a number of strategies to overcome this difficulty, including expressing different family members of nAChR or its sub-domain (mostly ECD), constructing AChBP-nAChR chimera, and introducing specific mutations to enhance expression and stability [32]. Using the nAChR $\alpha1$ as an example, we screened a PCR-generated mutant library of mouse nAChR $\alpha1$ ECD for variants with increased expression and stability which led to the isolation of a triple mutant (V8E/W149R/V155A) that has much improved expression and stability than the wild type protein, and ultimately the determination of the crystal structure of nAChR $\alpha1$ ECD bound to a-bungarotoxin at 1.94 Å resolution [22]. Structure comparison with the 4 Å electron microscopic model of nAChR and AChBP reveals that the isolated ECD is very similar to its counterpart in the intact channel and that the stabilizing mutations do not appear to alter the overall structure of the ECD.

All of the three mutations map to the surface of the protein (**Figure 1a**), with one (V8E) located on the N-terminal helix and the other two (W149R and V155A) located on loop B. The V8E mutation introduces a salt bridge with Lys84 (**Figure 1b**), whereas the W149R mutation introduces a salt bridge with Asp89 (**Figure 1c**). These salt bridges apparently contribute to protein stability as evident by the well-defined electron density of these exposed residues with long and charged side chains. Thus, the mutations seem to enhance the protein stability through at least two mechanisms. One is to remove surface exposed hydrophobic residues, including V155A (**Figure 1d**); the other is to introduce salt bridges on the protein surface. These observations suggest that the ECD of nAChR may be rationally engineered to improve solubility and stability. In principle, one can use homology models to guide the selection of exposed hydrophobic residues and to engineer surface salt bridges, which can increase the stability of recombinant mammalian nAChRs. This insight will be important for the design of stable chimeric nAChR antigen for specific targeting and elimination of nAChR-specific B cells (discussed further below).

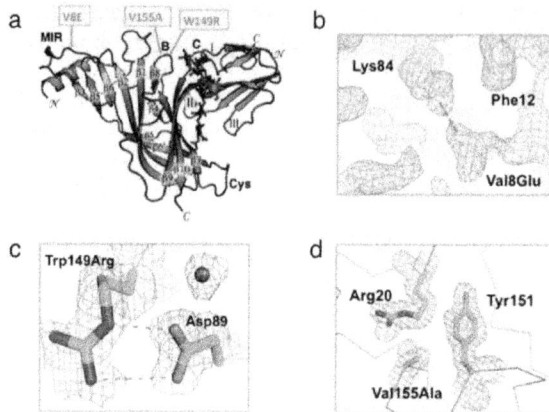

Figure 1.
Mutations that stabilize nAChR α1 ECD. (a) The three mutations (boxed and indicated by arrow) are mapped on the surface of nAChR α1 ECD (dark green) and away from the binding site of α-bungarotoxin (orange) and the glycan (magenta); (b) the mutation Val8Glu establishes a salt bridge with Lys84. The surrounding structure is well ordered, showing well-defined electron density; (c) the mutation Trp149Arg establishes a salt bridge with Asp89. The side chains of both residues show well-defined electron density; (d) the mutation of Val155Ala removes an exposed hydrophobic residue. The surrounding structure is well ordered (Adapted from Chen [33]).

4. Functionally instrinsic instability of nAChR ECD

Most proteins have a densely packed hydrophobic core that is important for stable folding in aqueous solution. However, a hydration pocket was found inside the beta sandwich core of the nAChR α1 ECD [22]. This hydration pocket consists of two buried hydrophilic residues, Thr52 and Ser126, two ordered water molecules, and a few cavities, creating a packing defect near the disulfide that connects the two beta sheets. Both Thr52 and Ser126 are highly conserved in nAChRs but are substituted by large hydrophobic residues (Phe, Leu or Val) in the non-channel homologue AChBPs. This observation suggests that the nAChR ECD has evolved with a non-optimally packed core, hence predisposed to undergo conformational change during ligand-induced gating. Replacing Thr52 and Ser126 with their hydrophobic counterparts in AChBP significantly impaired the gating function of nAChR without affecting the folding of the protein structure [22]. This role of the hydration pocket on the conformation flexibility/dynamics of the nAChR ECD is supported by recent molecular dynamics studies [34]. This model also suggests that the specific location of the hydration cavity is important for a particular class of pentameric LGICs [35]. A practical implication of these observations is that one can design stabilization mutants of LGICs, including nAChR ECD, by structure-guided modifications of such packing defects, which are evolved for intrinsic ion channel functions but may be detrimental to recombinant production of proteins as therapeutic antigen.

5. Structural studies of the complexes between nAChR ECD and EAMG antibodies

Antibodies generated by the immune system may bind various epitopes on nAChR. It is therefore important to know if MG autoantibodies are randomly distributed to various epitopes and if they contribute equally or differently to the disease phenotype. This question is also therapeutically relevant if one wishes to use small molecules or single valent antibody [36] to block the binding of most pathologically relevant autoantibodies to nAChR. Mammalian muscle nAChR has a pentameric structure composed of two α1, one β1, one δ, and one ε (adult form) or γ (fetal form) subunit(s) [18]. Extensive studies suggest that autoantibodies to α1 play a major role in MG pathology [37–40]. Furthermore, more than half of all autoantibodies in MG and EAMG bind an overlapping region on the nAChR α1 subunit, known as the main immunogenic region (MIR) [41]. The MIR is defined by the ability of a single rat monoclonal antibody (mAb), mAb35, to inhibit the binding of about 65% autoantibodies from MG patients or rats with EAMG [42–44]. Subsequent studies have mapped MIR to a peptide region that spans residues 67–76 on nAChR α1 [45, 46]. Monoclonal antibodies directed to the MIR can passively transfer EAMG and possess all the key pathological functions of serum autoantibodies from MG patients [37]. Moreover, a recent study showed that titer levels of MIR-competing autoantibodies from MG patients, rather than the total amount of nAChR autoantibodies, correlate with disease severity [47]. These observations suggest that autoantibodies directed to the MIR on nAChR α1 play a major role in the pathogenesis of MG [41]. However, autoantibodies classified as MIR-directed by competition assay may not necessarily have the same binding mechanisms to nAChR: two MIR-competing autoantibodies may share common or overlapping epitopes or may bind different epitopes but compete through steric effect [14].

Given their established myasthenogenic role, extensive efforts have been put into characterizing the interactions between MG autoantibodies and nAChR using biochemical [45, 46, 48–53], structural [22, 54–56], and modeling approaches [57]. More recently, the first crystal structures of human (pdb code: 5HBT) and mouse (pdb code: 5HBV) nAChR ECD bound by the Fab fragment of an EAMG autoantibody, Fab35 were determined [58]. Both crystal structures are very similar, so the discussion here will focus mainly on the human complex (pdb code: 5HBT). The crystal structure, which also contains α-Btx that binds and stabilizes nAChR ECD to facilitate crystallization, shows that Fab35 binds to nAChR α1 in an upright orientation, away from the α-Btx (**Figure 2**). The Fab35 binding sites on nAChR α1 include the MIR and the N-terminal helix. Fab35 has the canonical IgG antibody structure where the complementarity determining regions (CDRs) from the heavy chain, CDR-H2 and CDR-H3, and the light chain, CDR-L3, form the binding site for nAChR α1. Contacting residues from Fab35 and nAChR α1 (defined as being closer than 4.5 Å) can be mapped using the crystal structure. Such contacting analysis revealed several "hotspots" on nAChR α1 that make numerous contacts to Fab35, including Asn68 and Asp71 from the MIR loop and Arg6 and Lys10 from the N-terminal helix. As shown in **Figure 3**, each of these four "hotspots" anchors an extensive network of interactions that display remarkable chemical complementarities. The importance of these hotspots are supported by extensive mutagenesis studies [50, 51, 53, 59], which showed that Asn68 and Asp71 of the MIR are essential for MG autoantibody binding, while the surrounding Pro69 and Tyr72, when mutated, also affect the interaction between the antibody and the receptor. Mutation of N68D and D71K in the intact receptor also suggested ASn68 and Asp71 are of vital importance for the interaction [49]. On the N-terminal helix of *Torpedo* nAChR α1, two exposed residues, Arg6 and Asn10, which correspond to Arg6 and Lys10 in human nAChR α1, respectively, are found to be critical to MG antibody binding by mutational analyses [53]. Many nAChR residues found to be important for antibody binding by mutagenesis studies, including Asn68 and Asp71of the MIR and Arg6 and Lys10 of the N-terminal helix, were indeed found to be interaction "hotspots" at the Fab35/nAChR α1 interface. More recent studies using natively folded nAChR α1α7 chimera proteins [52] or GFP-fused protein fragments [53] showed that the N-terminal helix (residues 1–14) and the nearby loop region (residues 15–32) are also important for high affinity MG antibody binding. These biochemical observations are in excellent agreement with the binding interface structure observed in the crystals (**Figure 2**).

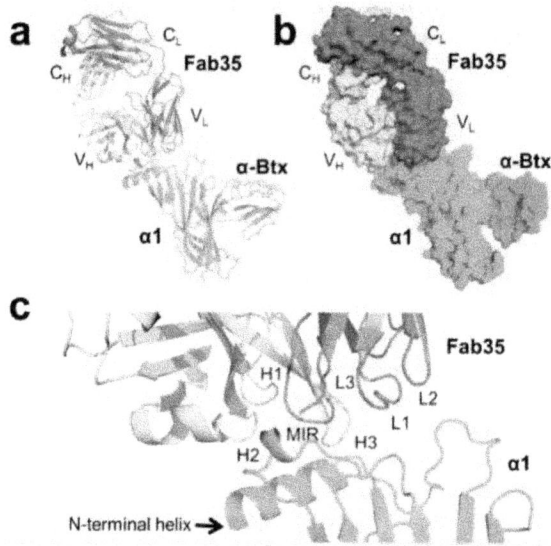

Figure 2.
Crystal structure of the ternary complex of nAChR α1 ECD bound by Fab35 and α-Btx. (a) Ribbon representation of nAChR α1 ECD (α1: cyan) in complex with α-Btx (green) and Fab35 (heavy chain (H, yellow) and light chain (L, magenta)). The variable domains (VH and VL) and the constant domains (CH and CL) of the antibody are indicated accordingly. (b) Surface representation of the ternary complex. (c) Zoomed-in view of the binding interface. The complementarity determining regions of the heavy chain and light chain are indicated as H1, H2, H3, L1, L2, and L3, respectively (Adapted from Noridomi et al. [58]).

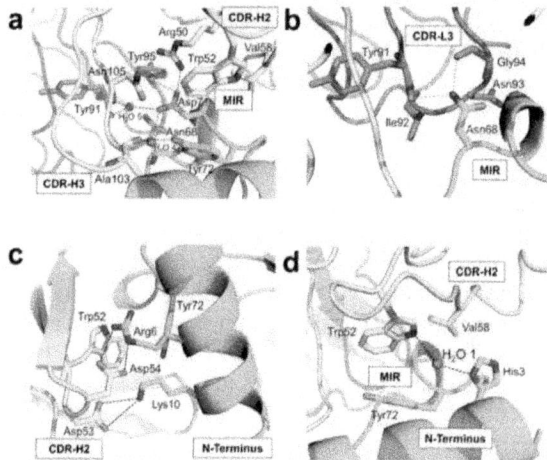

Figure 3.
Detailed interactions between Fab35 and nAChR α1 ECD at the binding interface. (a) Binding interactions at the vicinity of Asp71 of α1 (located at the MIR). (b) Interactions at the vicinity of Asn68 of α1 (located at the MIR). (c) Interactions involving Arg6 and Lys10 of α1 (located at the N-terminus of α1). (d) Interactions mediated by His3 of α1 (located at the N-terminus of α1) (Adapted from Noridomi et al. [58]).

Although biochemical mapping of antibody-binding residues on nAChR α1 were performed with different antibodies (e.g., mAb210 and mAb132A) [45, 46, 48–53], it is remarkable that these biochemical data agree so well with the crystal structure. The fact that many MIR residues at the center of the antibody-receptor interface are important for the high affinity binding of a variety of MG antibodies suggests that many MIR-directed autoantibodies share similar binding mechanisms to the core MIR/N-helix region. This is a rather surprising finding given the potential heterogeneity of nAChR antibodies mentioned above. An important implication of this finding is that it may be possible to find small molecule inhibitors to block the binding of a large fraction of pathological MG autoantibodies to nAChR.

6. Structural comparison of Fab35 with other MG autoantibodies

To see how various MG/EAMG mAbs may bind nAChR through similar or different mechanisms, we compared the structure of Fab35 with that of two other MG mAbs (Fab198: pdb code 1FN4 and Fab192: pdb code, 1C5D) that have been determined previously [55, 56]. Superposition of the structure of Fab198 and Fab35 from the ternary complex shows that these two Fabs share a similar antigen-binding site (**Figure 4a**). As such, the MIR loop fits snugly into the pocket formed by the CDR-H2, CDR-H3 and CDR-L3 loops of Fab198, as predicated by previous modeling studies [57]. The CDR-H2 loop of Fab198 is also in a position to interact with the N-terminal α-helix adjacent to the MIR (**Figure 4b**). Even more remarkably, many key α1-binding residues in Fab35 are also conserved in Fab198 and they appear to have similar contacts to nAChR α1 in the modeled Fab198/nAChR α1 binding interface (**Figure 4b**). These residues include Trp47 from CDR-H2, Arg50 from CDR-H2, and Tyr95 from CDR-L3 at the center of the MIR-binding pocket, and Trp52 and Asp54 (both from CDR-H2) which interact with the N-terminal α-helix. In contrast to the structural similarities shown above, the CDR-H3 loops between Fab198 and Fab35 differ significantly in length and sequence. The CDR-H3 loop of Fab198 is too short to interact with the surface pocket of nAChR α1, which is occupied by the corresponding CDR-H3 loop of Fab35 in the complex crystal structure (**Figure 4b**). These structural analyses suggest that mAb35 and mAb198 share a high degree of similarity in binding mechanism to the core MIR/N-terminal helix region but differ in the periphery of the binding interface. On the other hand, superposition of the structure of Fab192 onto that of Fab35 in the ternary complex reveals substantial differences (not shown here). The variable domains (V_H and V_L) have a significant rotational twist, such that the MIR loop does not fit into the antigen-binding site of Fab192. What is more, the key α1-binding residues of Fab35, like Arg50 and Trp52 of CDR-H2, are not conserved in Fab192. These structural differences suggest that Fab192 may differ significantly from Fab35 in terms of binding mechanisms to nAChR α1, confirming and extending the differences previously recognized between the two [52].

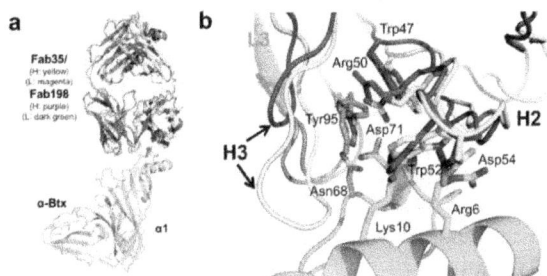

Figure 4.
Structural comparisons among MG mAbs. (a) Superposition of Fab198 [55] (heavy chain: purple and light chain: dark green) onto Fab35 in the Fab35/nAChR α1/α-Btx ternary complex using the Cα backbone. (b) Detailed comparison of the binding interface. The residues are colored according to their protein subunits.

7. MG autoantibody repertoire and MIR-directed autoantibodies

A number of studies showed that the total amount of nAChR antibodies in the serum of MG patients does not seem to correlate with disease severity, suggesting that various nAChR antibodies that bind different regions on nAChR may contribute differently to this disease [41, 60–62]. As discussed above, the total amount of autoantibody from MG patients directed to the MIR of nAChR α1 subunit did show significant correlation with disease severity [47]. These observations suggest that autoantibodies directed to nAChR α1 MIR play a major role in the pathogenesis of MG [41]. It is now clear that many MIR-directed autoantibodies bind a composite epitope consisting of the original MIR (α1, 67–76) and the N-terminal helix (α1, 2–14) (N-helix) and surrounding regions (α1, 15–32). The structural analyses above and published biochemical data suggest that some MIR-directed autoantibodies (e.g., mAb35 and mAb198) bind epitopes centered around the MIR/N-helix core region while others (e.g., mAb192) seems to require epitopes outside the MIR/N-helix core. Nevertheless, based on crystallography studies and structure-guided analyses of existing biochemical data, it can be concluded that despite the heterogeneity of MG autoantibody repertoire a large fraction of MG autoantibodies share a highly-conserved binding mechanism to a core region on the nAChR, suggesting that it is possible to use a single or a limited set of small molecules to block the binding of a large fraction of MG autoantibodies. Because MG autoantibodies directed to the MIR region on nAChR are most relevant to the MG disease, MIR and its surrounding region are therefore an attractive target site for developing small molecules to block the binding of MG autoantibodies. Blocking the binding of MG autoantibodies to nAChR will likely have a direct impact on the antibody-mediated pathologies and may even alter the long-term immune response to nAChR in MG patient.

8. Small molecules blocking the binding of MIR-directed autoantibody to nAChR

Targeting protein-protein interface for drug development is generally more challenging than the enzyme active sites [63]. This is especially true for flat protein interfaces lacking features for small molecule binding. However, successes have been achieved with a number of well-known targets, including the p53/MDM2 complex [64], the Bcl-xL/Bak complex [65] and the IL2/IL2R complex [66, 67]. A common feature of these complexes is that the protein-protein binding interfaces contain concave pockets lined with hydrophobic residues, which may provide favorable anchoring points for small molecules to bind and compete with protein-protein interactions. The crystal structure of the Fab35/nAChR α1 complex revealed that their binding interface is characterized by mutual insertions of loops into the pockets of binding partners. On the receptor side (**Figure 5**), the MIR loop inserts deeply into a surface pocket between V_H and V_L, and the N-terminal α-helix sits into a groove on the surface of V_H. On the antibody side (**Figure 6**), the CDR-H3 protrudes into a surface pocket formed by the N-terminal α-helix, the loop following the N-terminal α-helix, the MIR and the loop preceding the MIR (referred to as the CDRH3 pocket here after). Based on these structural features, two MG inhibitor design strategies can be envisioned. One is to find small molecules that bind the surface pockets on Fab35 (**Figure 5**). But this approach faces the potential issue of antibody heterogeneity in sera of human MG patients because small molecule inhibitors may bind some but not other pathological autoantibodies, as it is highly possible antibodies binding to the same epitope may have subtle differences in their antigen-binding site structures. Another approach is to find small molecules to bind the CDRH3 pocket on nAChR (**Figure 6**). Small molecules bound to this site will directly interfere with the binding

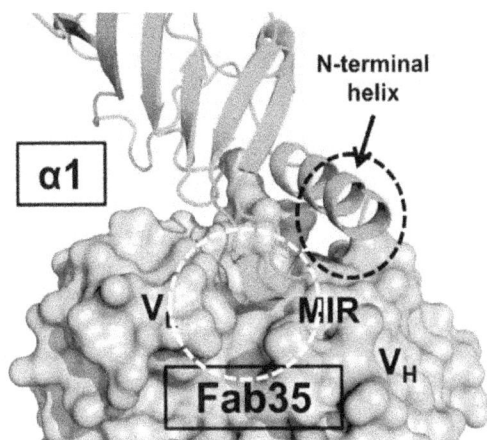

Figure 5.
Surface pockets on Fab35 bound by the nAChR MIR loop (white dashed circle) and the N-terminal helix (black dashed circle).

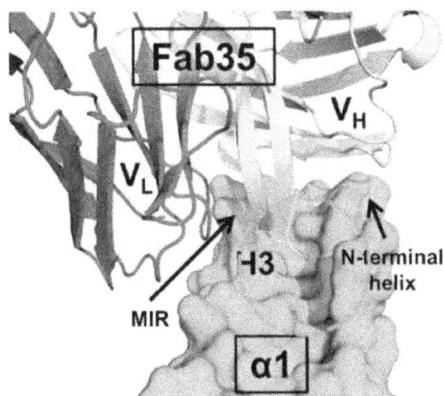

Figure 6.
The surface pocket (green dashed circle) on nAChR α1 bound by the CDR-H3 loop from Fab35 (indicated as H3 in the figure).

of mAB35 by competing with its CDR-H3. Even for other mAbs with short CDR-H3, such as mAb198, the compounds may also block the binding of CDR-H3 through steric hindrances. Moreover, since the CDRH3 pocket is immediate adjacent (about 6–8 Å) (**Figure 6**) to the MIR/N-helix core region critical for the binding of a large group of MG autoantibodies, compounds bound to CDRH3 could sterically and/or allosterically inhibit the binding of most pathological MG autoantibodies efficiently. Because of its concaved structure, CDRH3 pocket could serve as the anchoring point to design and/or screen small molecules that bind nAChR α1 and complete with MG autoantibodies directed to MIR and its nearby regions.

9. nAChR-specific B cell inhibition and depletion with engineered antigen chimera

The fact that pathogenic B cell clones can populate for a long time in patients' body may explain why MG is usually a chronic disease. Ectopic germinal centers are found in the thymus of many MG patients who are diagnosed with thymoma or thymus hyperplasia, where nAChR-specific B lymphocyte are constantly activated, selected and matured to produce the antibody, leading to the disease [68]. This disease model underlies the rationale of thymectomy as a widely adopted treatment of MG, but the result varies depending on the subtype of the disease, with a complete remission rate of 25–53% [69]. These results suggest there are possibly other unknown sites where nAChR specific B cells are activated, selected and matured [13].

Using B cell surface marker CD20 [70–72] or possibly CD19 [73] as the target, disease-causing B cells can be depleted at the cost of killing normal B cells. For example, an ongoing clinical trial, NCT02110706, is testing if rituximab, which targets CD20 on B cells, can be a safe and beneficial therapeutics for MG. In general, treatment with B cell depletion agent often requires a long recovery time before B cells return to normal level again [71]. Moreover, the treatment has been reported to have a short effective duration time for MuSK-positive MG [74]. Long-term usage of such agent may compromise immunological function with increased risk of infection such as Progressive multifocal leukoencephalopathy (PML) and malignancy [72]. As such, strategies targeting nAChR specific B cells seem to be attractive. Since each B cell expresses B cell Receptors of the same idiotype as its secreted antibody on its surface, one can use such property to specifically target autoreactive B cell as long as the antigenicity of the autoimmune disease is clear. The idea was borrowed from immunotoxins [75] in which an antigen-toxin chimera was constructed. The antigen moiety is used to target the B cells that express the BCR of the same idiotype as the antibody and the toxin moiety is responsible for conveying death signal to the target B cells. In a pioneering study in 1983 the author fused thymoglobulin with ricin to treat an autoimmune disorder-Hashimoto's thyroiditis [76]. Another attempt was tried a decade later in another autoimmune disease-Pemphigus Vulgaris, in which the authors constructed antigen-toxin fusion protein that can specifically target Dsg3-specific hybridoma cells [77]. Similar strategies have also been attempted in the treatment of MG. In a study of 2006, the author fused the nAChR α1 ECD to a plant toxin and showed its effectiveness in specifically killing of α1-specific B cells [78]. More recently, researchers have developed a variant of such strategy in which nAChR α1 ECD was fused with Fc domain of antibody, which was used to convey the negative signal, since B cells express and only express one kind of Fc receptor, namely FcRγIIB, which transduce negative signal for B cell activation. Consequently, such chimeric protein will specifically target the nAChR α1 specific B cell via the binding to the BCR and deliver negative signal to inhibit α1 specific B cells [79, 80].

The idea of antigen-chimera in the treatment of MG seems attractive but will not be practical unless the chimeric protein is stable enough to be used as a therapeutic agent. As mentioned above, nAChR α1 is just one subunit of the nAChR pentamer and is intrinsically unstable, making the expression of wild type nAChR α1 ECD in stable soluble form very challenging. However, as discussed earlier in this chapter, crystallography studies of nAChR α1 ECD in recent years have accumulated extensive experience and knowledge in designing strategic mutations to improve the stability and expression level of nAChR α1 ECD protein while preserve the binding of MIR-directed MG autoantibodies [22, 31, 58] These progresses will greatly facilitate the approach to using engineered antigen chimera to specially inhibit and eliminate nAChR-specific B cells for MG treatment.

10. Outlook

Insights from structural studies and molecular biology/biochemical analyses may ultimately lead to precision medicine and personalized treatment of MG by antigen profiling of patient and the use of corresponding molecular missiles to eliminate antigen specific antibodies or B-cells, induce antigen specific tolerance, or blocking nAChR-autoantibody binding by small molecules. These approaches, once established in the treatment of MG, could be expanded to other autoimmune diseases with well-defined antigen targets.

Author details

Jiang Xu, Kaori Noridomi and Lin Chen*
Molecular and Computational Biology, Departments of Biological Sciences and Chemistry, University of Southern California, Los Angeles, CA, USA

*Address all correspondence to: linchen@usc.edu

IntechOpen

References

[1] Philips L. The epidemiology of myasthenia gravis. Annals of the New York Academy of Sciences. 2003;**998**:407-412. DOI: 10.1196/annals.1254.053

[2] Hoch W, McConville J, Helms S, Newsom-Davis J, Melms A, Vincent A. Auto-antibodies to the receptor tyrosine kinase MuSK in patients with myasthenia gravis without acetylcholine receptor antibodies. Nature Medicine. 2001;**7**:365. DOI: 10.1038/85520

[3] Zhang B, Tzartos JS, Belimezi M, Ragheb S, Bealmear B, Lewis RA, et al. Autoantibodies to lipoprotein-related protein 4 in patients with double-seronegative myasthenia gravis. Archives of Neurology. 2012;**69**:445-451. DOI: 10.1001/archneurol.2011.2393

[4] Vincent A, Palace J, Hilton-Jones D. Myasthenia gravis. Lancet (London, England). 2001;**357**:2122-2128. DOI: 10.1016/S0140-6736(00)05186-2

[5] Gomez AM, Vrolix K, Martínez-Martínez P, Molenaar PC, Phernambucq M, van der Esch E, et al. Proteasome inhibition with bortezomib depletes plasma cells and autoantibodies in experimental autoimmune myasthenia gravis. Journal of Immunology. 2011;**186**:2503-2513. DOI: 10.4049/JIMMUNOL.1002539

[6] Gomez AM, Willcox N, Molenaar PC, Buurman W, Martinez-Martinez P, De Baets MH, et al. Targeting plasma cells with proteasome inhibitors: Possible roles in treating myasthenia gravis? Annals of the New York Academy of Sciences. 2012;**1274**:48-59. DOI: 10.1111/j.1749-6632.2012.06824.x

[7] Gold R, Dalakas MC, Toyka KV. Immunotherapy in autoimmune neuromuscular disorders. Lancet Neurology. 2003;**2**:22-32. DOI: 10.1016/S1474-4422(03)00264-3

[8] Nicolle MW, Nag B, Sharma SD, Willcox N, Vincent A, Ferguson DJ, et al. Specific tolerance to an acetylcholine receptor epitope induced in vitro in myasthenia gravis CD4+ lymphocytes by soluble major histocompatibility complex class II-peptide complexes. The Journal of Clinical Investigation. 1994;**93**:1361-1369. DOI: 10.1172/JCI117112

[9] Okumura S, McIntosh K, Drachman DB. Oral administration of acetylcholine receptor: Effects on experimental myasthenia gravis. Annals of Neurology. 1994;**36**:704-713. DOI: 10.1002/ana.410360504

[10] Karachunski PI, Ostlie NS, Okita DK, Garman R, Conti-Fine BM. Subcutaneous administration of T-epitope sequences of the acetylcholine receptor prevents experimental myasthenia gravis. Journal of Neuroimmunology. 1999;**93**:108-121. DOI: 10.1016/S0165-5728(98)00208-2

[11] Pass-Rozner M, Faber-Elmann A, Sela M, Mozes E. Immunomodulation of myasthenia gravis associated autoimmune responses by an altered peptide ligand: Mechanisms of action. In: Myasthenia gravis. Dordrecht: Springer Netherlands; 2000. pp. 182-194. DOI: 10.1007/978-94-011-4060-7_17

[12] Wu B, Goluszko E, Christadoss P. Experimental autoimmune myasthenia gravis in the mouse. In: Current Protocols in Immunology. Hoboken, NJ, USA: John Wiley & Sons, Inc.; 2001. pp. 15.8.1-15.8.19. DOI: 10.1002/0471142735.im1508s21

[13] Yi H-J, Chae C-S, So J-S, Tzartos SJ, Souroujon MC, Fuchs S, et al. Suppression of experimental myasthenia gravis by a B-cell epitope-free recombinant acetylcholine receptor. Molecular Immunology.

2008;**46**:192-201. DOI: 10.1016/J.
MOLIMM.2008.08.264

[14] Luo J, Lindstrom J. AChR-specific
immunosuppressive therapy of
myasthenia gravis. Biochemical
Pharmacology. 2015;**97**:609-619. DOI:
10.1016/J.BCP.2015.07.011

[15] Hurst R, Rollema H, Bertrand D.
Nicotinic acetylcholine receptors: From
basic science to therapeutics. Pharmacology
& Therapeutics. 2013;**137**:22-54. DOI:
10.1016/J.PHARMTHERA.2012.08.012

[16] Sine SM, Engel AG. Recent advances
in Cys-loop receptor structure and
function. Nature. 2006;**440**:448-455.
DOI: 10.1038/nature04708

[17] Miyazawa A, Fujiyoshi Y, Unwin N.
Structure and gating mechanism of the
acetylcholine receptor pore. Nature.
2003;**423**:949-955. DOI: 10.1038/
nature01748

[18] Unwin N. Refined structure of the
nicotinic acetylcholine receptor at 4 Å
resolution. Journal of Molecular Biology.
2005;**346**:967-989. DOI: 10.1016/j.
jmb.2004.12.031

[19] Brejc K, van Dijk WJ, Klaassen RV,
Schuurmans M, van der Oost J, Smit AB,
et al. Crystal structure of an ACh-binding
protein reveals the ligand-binding
domain of nicotinic receptors. Nature.
2001;**411**:269-276. DOI: 10.1038/35077011

[20] Rucktooa P, Smit AB, Sixma TK.
Insight in nAChR subtype selectivity
from AChBP crystal structures.
Biochemical Pharmacology.
2009;**78**:777-787. DOI: 10.1016/J.
BCP.2009.06.098

[21] Karlin A. A touching picture
of nicotinic binding. Neuron.
2004;**41**:841-842. DOI: 10.1016/
S0896-6273(04)00151-5

[22] Dellisanti CD, Yao Y, Stroud JC,
Wang Z-Z, Chen L. Crystal structure

of the extracellular domain of nAChR
α1 bound to α-bungarotoxin at 1.94 Å
resolution. Nature Neuroscience.
2007;**10**:953-962. DOI: 10.1038/nn1942

[23] Hilf RJC, Dutzler R. X-ray
structure of a prokaryotic pentameric
ligand-gated ion channel. Nature.
2008;**452**:375-379. DOI: 10.1038/
nature06717

[24] Hilf RJC, Dutzler R. Structure of
a potentially open state of a proton-
activated pentameric ligand-gated ion
channel. Nature. 2009;**457**:115-118.
DOI: 10.1038/nature07461

[25] Bocquet N, Nury H, Baaden M, Le
Poupon C, Changeux J-P, Delarue M,
et al. X-ray structure of a pentameric
ligand-gated ion channel in an
apparently open conformation. Nature.
2009;**457**:111-114. DOI: 10.1038/
nature07462

[26] Corringer P-J, Poitevin F, Prevost MS,
Sauguet L, Delarue M, Changeux J-P.
Structure and pharmacology of
pentameric receptor channels:
From bacteria to brain. Structure.
2012;**20**:941-956. DOI: 10.1016/J.
STR.2012.05.003

[27] Hibbs RE, Gouaux E. Principles of
activation and permeation in an anion-
selective Cys-loop receptor. Nature.
2011;**474**:54-60. DOI: 10.1038/nature10139

[28] Morales-Perez CL, Noviello CM, Hibbs
RE. X-ray structure of the human α4β2
nicotinic receptor. Nature. 2016;**538**:
411-415. DOI: 10.1038/nature19785

[29] Taly A, Corringer P-J, Guedin D,
Lestage P, Changeux J-P. Nicotinic
receptors: Allosteric transitions and
therapeutic targets in the nervous
system. Nature Reviews. Drug
Discovery. 2009;**8**:733-750. DOI:
10.1038/nrd2927

[30] Psaridi-Linardaki L, Mamalaki A,
Remoundos M, Tzartos SJ. Expression

of soluble ligand- and antibody-binding extracellular domain of human muscle acetylcholine receptor alpha subunit in yeast *Pichia pastoris*. Role of glycosylation in alpha-bungarotoxin binding. The Journal of Biological Chemistry. 2002;**277**:26980-26986. DOI: 10.1074/jbc.M110731200

[31] Yao Y, Wang J, Viroonchatapan N, Samson A, Chill J, Rothe E, et al. Yeast expression and NMR analysis of the extracellular domain of muscle nicotinic acetylcholine receptor alpha subunit. The Journal of Biological Chemistry. 2002;**277**:12613-12621. DOI: 10.1074/jbc.M108845200

[32] Zouridakis M, Zisimopoulou P, Poulas K, Tzartos SJ. Recent advances in understanding the structure of nicotinic acetylcholine receptors. IUBMB Life. 2009;**61**:407-423. DOI: 10.1002/iub.170

[33] Chen L. In pursuit of the high-resolution structure of nicotinic acetylcholine receptors. The Journal of Physiology. 2010;**588**:557-564. DOI: 10.1113/jphysiol.2009.184085

[34] Cheng X, Ivanov I, Wang H, Sine SM, McCammon JA. Molecular-dynamics simulations of ELIC—A prokaryotic homologue of the nicotinic acetylcholine receptor. Biophysical Journal. 2009;**96**:4502-4513. DOI: 10.1016/J.BPJ.2009.03.018

[35] Dellisanti CD, Hanson SM, Chen L, Czajkowski C. Packing of the extracellular domain hydrophobic core has evolved to facilitate pentameric ligand-gated ion channel function. The Journal of Biological Chemistry. 2011;**286**:3658-3670. DOI: 10.1074/jbc.M110.156851

[36] Tsantili P, Tzartos SJ, Mamalaki A. High affinity single-chain Fv antibody fragments protecting the human nicotinic acetylcholine receptor. Journal of Neuroimmunology. 1999;**94**:15-27. DOI: 10.1016/S0165-5728(98)00195-7

[37] Tzartos S, Hochschwender S, Vasquez P, Lindstrom J. Passive transfer of experimental autoimmune myasthenia gravis by monoclonal antibodies to the main immunogenic region of the acetylcholine receptor. Journal of Neuroimmunology. 1987;**15**:185-194. DOI: 10.1016/0165-5728(87)90092-0

[38] Sideris S, Lagoumintzis G, Kordas G, Kostelidou K, Sotiriadis A, Poulas K, et al. Isolation and functional characterization of anti-acetylcholine receptor subunit-specific autoantibodies from myasthenic patients: Receptor loss in cell culture. Journal of Neuroimmunology. 2007;**189**:111-117. DOI: 10.1016/J.JNEUROIM.2007.06.014

[39] Tzartos SJ, Bitzopoulou K, Gavra I, Kordas G, Jacobson L, Kostelidou K, et al. Antigen-specific apheresis of pathogenic autoantibodies from myasthenia gravis sera. Annals of the New York Academy of Sciences. 2008;**1132**:291-299. DOI: 10.1196/annals.1405.017

[40] Kordas G, Lagoumintzis G, Sideris S, Poulas K, Tzartos SJ. Direct proof of the in vivo pathogenic role of the AChR autoantibodies from myasthenia gravis patients. PLoS One. 2014;**9**:e108327. DOI: 10.1371/journal.pone.0108327

[41] Tzartos SJ, Barkas T, Cung MT, Mamalaki A, Marraud M, Orlewski P, et al. Anatomy of the antigenic structure of a large memberane autoantigen, the muscle-type nicotinic acetylcholine receptor. Immunological Reviews. 1998;**163**:89-120. DOI: 10.1111/j.1600-065X.1998.tb01190.x

[42] Tzartos SJ, Lindstrom JM. Monoclonal antibodies used to probe acetylcholine receptor structure: Localization of the main immunogenic region and detection of similarities between subunits. Proceedings of the National Academy of Sciences.

1980;**77**:755-759. DOI: 10.1073/PNAS.77.2.755

[43] Tzartos SJ, Seybold ME, Lindstrom JM. Specificities of antibodies to acetylcholine receptors in sera from myasthenia gravis patients measured by monoclonal antibodies. Proceedings of the National Academy of Sciences of the United States of America. 1982;**79**:188. https://www.ncbi.nlm.nih.gov/pmc/articles/PMC345688/ [Accessed: December 27, 2018]

[44] Tzartos S, Langeberg L, Hochschwender S, Lindstrom J. Demonstration of a main immunogenic region on acetylcholine receptors from human muscle using monoclonal antibodies to human receptor. FEBS Letters. 1983;**158**:116-118. DOI: 10.1016/0014-5793(83)80688-7

[45] Barkas T, Gabriel JM, Mauron A, Hughes GJ, Roth B, Alliod C, et al. Monoclonal antibodies to the main immunogenic region of the nicotinic acetylcholine receptor bind to residues 61-76 of the alpha subunit. The Journal of Biological Chemistry. 1988;**263**:5916-5920. http://www.ncbi.nlm.nih.gov/pubmed/2451673 [Accessed: December 27, 2018]

[46] Tzartos SJ, Kokla A, Walgrave SL, Conti-Tronconi BM. Localization of the main immunogenic region of human muscle acetylcholine receptor to residues 67-76 of the alpha subunit. Proceedings of the National Academy of Sciences of the United States of America. 1988;**85**:2899-2903. http://www.ncbi.nlm.nih.gov/pubmed/3362855 [Accessed: December 27, 2018]

[47] Masuda T, Motomura M, Utsugisawa K, Nagane Y, Nakata R, Tokuda M, et al. Antibodies against the main immunogenic region of the acetylcholine receptor correlate with disease severity in myasthenia gravis.

Journal of Neurology, Neurosurgery, and Psychiatry. 2012;**83**:935-940. DOI: 10.1136/jnnp-2012-302705

[48] Das MK, Lindstrom J. The main immunogenic region of the nicotinic acetylcholine receptor: Interaction of monoclonal antibodies with synthetic peptides. Biochemical and Biophysical Research Communications. 1989;**165**:865-871. DOI: 10.1016/S0006-291X(89)80046-4

[49] Saedi MS, Anand R, Conroy WG, Lindstrom J. Determination of amino acids critical to the main immunogenic region of intact acetylcholine receptors by in vitro mutagenesis. FEBS Letters. 1990;**267**:55-59. DOI: 10.1016/0014-5793(90)80286-R

[50] Papadouli I, Potamianos S, Hadjidakis I, Bairaktari E, Tsikaris V, Sakarellos C, et al. Antigenic role of single residues within the main immunogenic region of the nicotinic acetylcholine receptor. The Biochemical Journal. 1990;**269**:239-245. DOI: 10.1042/BJ2690239

[51] Papadouli I, Sakarellos C, Tzartos SJ. High-resolution epitope mapping and fine antigenic characterization of the main immunogenic region of the acetylcholine receptor: Improving the binding activity of synthetic analogues of the region. European Journal of Biochemistry. 1993;**211**:227-234. DOI: 10.1111/j.1432-1033.1993.tb19890.x

[52] Luo J, Taylor P, Losen M, De Baets MH, Shelton GD, Lindstrom J. Neurobiology of disease main immunogenic region structure promotes binding of conformation-dependent myasthenia gravis autoantibodies, nicotinic acetylcholine receptor conformation maturation, and agonist sensitivity. 2009;**29**(44):13898-13908. DOI: 10.1523/JNEUROSCI.2833-09.2009

[53] Morell SW, Trinh VB, Gudipati E, Friend A, Page NA, Agius MA, et al.

Structural characterization of the main immunogenic region of the Torpedo acetylcholine receptor. Molecular Immunology. 2014;**58**:116-131. DOI: 10.1016/J.MOLIMM.2013.11.005

[54] Beroukhim R, Unwin N. Three-dimensional location of the main immunogenic region of the acetylcholine receptor. Neuron. 1995;**15**:323-331. DOI: 10.1016/0896-6273(95)90037-3

[55] Kontou M, Leonidas DD, Vatzaki EH, Tsantili P, Mamalaki A, Oikonomakos NG, et al. The crystal structure of the Fab fragment of a rat monoclonal antibody against the main immunogenic region of the human muscle acetylcholine receptor. European Journal of Biochemistry. 2000;**267**:2389-2397. DOI: 10.1046/j.1432-1327.2000.01252.x

[56] Poulas K, Eliopoulos E, Vatzaki E, Navaza J, Kontou M, Oikonomakos N, et al. Crystal structure of Fab198, an efficient protector of the acetylcholine receptor against myasthenogenic antibodies. European Journal of Biochemistry. 2001;**268**:3685-3693. DOI: 10.1046/j.1432-1327.2001.02274.x

[57] Kleinjung J, Petit M-C, Orlewski P, Mamalaki A, Tzartos SJ, Tsikaris V, et al. The third-dimensional structure of the complex between an Fv antibody fragment and an analogue of the main immunogenic region of the acetylcholine receptor: A combined two-dimensional NMR, homology, and molecular modeling approach. Biopolymers. 2000;**53**: 113-128. DOI: 10.1002/(SICI)1097-0282(200002)53:2<113: AID-BIP1>3.0.CO;2-J

[58] Noridomi K, Watanabe G, Hansen MN, Han GW, Chen L. Structural insights into the molecular mechanisms of myasthenia gravis and their therapeutic implications. eLife. 2017;**6**. DOI: 10.7554/eLife.23043

[59] Bellone M, Tang F, Milius R, Conti-Tronconi BM. The main immunogenic region of the nicotinic acetylcholine receptor. Identification of amino acid residues interacting with different antibodies. Journal of Immunology. 1989;**143**:3568-3579. http://www.ncbi.nlm.nih.gov/pubmed/2584708 [Accessed: December 27, 2018]

[60] Mossman S, Vincent A, Newsom-Davis J. Passive transfer of myasthenia gravis by immunoglobulins: Lack of correlation between AChR with antibody bound, acetylcholine receptor loss and transmission defect. Journal of the Neurological Sciences. 1988;**84**:15-28. DOI: 10.1016/0022-510X(88)90170-0

[61] Somnier FE. Clinical implementation of anti-acetylcholine receptor antibodies. Journal of Neurology, Neurosurgery, and Psychiatry. 1993;**56**:496-504. http://www.ncbi.nlm.nih.gov/pubmed/8505642 [Accessed: December 27, 2018]

[62] Berrih-Aknin S. Myasthenia gravis, a model of organ-specific autoimmune disease. Journal of Autoimmunity. 1995;**8**:139-143. DOI: 10.1006/JAUT.1995.0011

[63] Scott DE, Bayly AR, Abell C, Skidmore J. Small molecules, big targets: Drug discovery faces the protein–protein interaction challenge. Nature Reviews. Drug Discovery. 2016;**15**: 533-550. DOI: 10.1038/nrd.2016.29

[64] Vassilev LT, Vu BT, Graves B, Carvajal D, Podlaski F, Filipovic Z, et al. In vivo activation of the p53 pathway by small-molecule antagonists of MDM2. Science. 2004;**303**:844-848. DOI: 10.1126/science.1092472

[65] Souers AJ, Leverson JD, Boghaert ER, Ackler SL, Catron ND, Chen J, et al. ABT-199, a potent and selective BCL-2 inhibitor, achieves antitumor activity while sparing platelets. Nature

Medicine. 2013;**19**:202-208. DOI: 10.1038/nm.3048

[66] Rickert M, Wang X, Boulanger MJ, Goriatcheva N, Garcia KC. The structure of interleukin-2 complexed with its alpha receptor. Science. 2005;**308**:1477-1480. DOI: 10.1126/science.1109745

[67] Wilson CGM, Arkin MR. Small-Molecule Inhibitors of IL-2/IL-2R: Lessons Learned and Applied. Berlin, Heidelberg: Springer; 2010. pp. 25-59. DOI: 10.1007/82_2010_93

[68] Sims GP, Shiono H, Willcox N, Stott DI. Somatic hypermutation and selection of B cells in thymic germinal centers responding to acetylcholine receptor in myasthenia gravis. Journal of Immunology. 2001;**167**:1935-1944. DOI: 10.4049/JIMMUNOL.167.4.1935

[69] Venuta F, Rendina EA, De Giacomo T, Della Rocca G, Antonini G, Ciccone AM, et al. Thymectomy for myasthenia gravis: A 27-year experience. European Journal of Cardio-Thoracic Surgery. 1999;**15**:621-624. Discussion 624-625. http://www.ncbi.nlm.nih.gov/pubmed/10386407 [Accessed: December 27, 2018]

[70] Dupuy A, Viguier M, Bédane C, Cordoliani F, Blaise S, Aucouturier F, et al. Treatment of refractory pemphigus vulgaris with rituximab (anti-CD20 monoclonal antibody). Archives of Dermatology. 2004;**140**: 91-96. DOI: 10.1001/archderm.140.1.91

[71] Yi JS, DeCroos EC, Sanders DB, Weinhold KJ, Guptill JT. Prolonged B-cell depletion in MuSK myasthenia gravis following rituximab treatment. Muscle & Nerve. 2013;**48**:992-993. DOI: 10.1002/mus.24063

[72] Du FH, Mills EA, Mao-Draayer Y. Next-generation anti-CD20 monoclonal antibodies in autoimmune disease treatment. Autoimmunity

Highlights. 2017;**8**:12. DOI: 10.1007/s13317-017-0100-y

[73] Chen D, Gallagher S, Monson N, Herbst R, Wang Y. Inebilizumab, a B cell-depleting anti-CD19 antibody for the treatment of autoimmune neurological diseases: Insights from preclinical studies. Journal of Clinical Medicine. 2016;**5**:107. DOI: 10.3390/jcm5120107

[74] Stathopoulos P, Kumar A, Nowak RJ, O'Connor KC. Autoantibody-producing plasmablasts after B cell depletion identified in muscle-specific kinase myasthenia gravis. JCI Insight. 2017;**2**(17):e94263 DOI: 10.1172/jci.insight.94263

[75] Madhumathi J, Verma RS. Therapeutic targets and recent advances in protein immunotoxins. Current Opinion in Microbiology. 2012;**15**:300-309. DOI: 10.1016/J.MIB.2012.05.006

[76] Rennie DP, McGregor AM, Wright J, Weetman AP, Hall R, Thorpe P. An immunotoxin of ricin A chain conjugated to thyroglobulin selectively suppresses the antithyroglobulin autoantibody response. Lancet (London, England). 1983;**2**:1338-1340. http://www.ncbi.nlm.nih.gov/pubmed/6139673 [Accessed: December 27, 2018]

[77] Proby CM, Ota T, Suzuki H, Koyasu S, Gamou S, Shimizu N, et al. Development of chimeric molecules for recognition and targeting of antigen-specific B cells in pemphigus vulgaris. The British Journal of Dermatology. 2000;**142**:321-330. DOI: 10.1046/j.1365-2133.2000.03328.x

[78] Hossann M, Li Z, Shi Y, Kreilinger U, Büttner J, Vogel PD, et al. Novel immunotoxin: A fusion protein consisting of gelonin and an acetylcholine receptor fragment as a potential immunotherapeutic agent for the treatment of Myasthenia gravis. Protein Expression and Purification.

2006;**46**:73-84. DOI: 10.1016/J. PEP.2005.08.029

[79] Chang T, Lin H, Gao J, Li W, Xu J, Sun CJ, et al. Selective recognition and elimination of nicotinic acetylcholine receptor-reactive B cells by a recombinant fusion protein AChR-Fc in myasthenia gravis in vitro. Journal of Neuroimmunology. 2010;**227**:35-43. DOI: 10.1016/j.jneuroim.2010.06.006

[80] Homma M, Uzawa A, Tanaka H, Kawaguchi N, Kanai T, Nakajima K, et al. A novel fusion protein, AChR-Fc, ameliorates myasthenia gravis by neutralizing antiacetylcholine receptor antibodies and suppressing acetylcholine receptor-reactive B cells. Neurotherapeutics. 2017;**14**:191-198. DOI: 10.1007/s13311-016-0476-9

Chapter 5

Plasmapheresis in Treatment of Myasthenia Gravis

Valerii Voinov

Abstract

Treatment of myasthenia gravis is still a rather difficult task, since there is no single tactic to use different drugs (corticosteroids, rituximab, immunoglobulins), especially since it is associated with a number of side effects. They are not able to remove the accumulating autoantibodies and immune complexes, the large size of which does not allow them to be excreted by the kidneys as well. Special problems of treatment arise when myasthenic crises develop associated with respiratory failure requiring artificial lungs ventilation. Plasmapheresis can help to solve this for it is possible to remove antibodies and other pathological metabolites. In addition, regular plasmapheresis is able not only to prevent exacerbations but also to reduce doses of the maintenance therapy with less risk of their side effects, which is confirmed by our own experience.

Keywords: myasthenia gravis, autoimmunity, autoantibodies, drug therapy, plasmapheresis

1. Introduction

Myasthenia gravis (MG) is a relatively rare disease, affecting about 140 people per million [1, 2]; however, its frequency has been increasing in the recent years, especially in the elderly population with mortality rate of 0.27/100,000 people, and in intensive care units, mortality of such patients reaches 5.3% [3, 4]. However, MG also affects children, manifesting in three forms: transient neonatal myasthenia, congenital myasthenic syndrome, and juvenile MG [5]. In the latter case, the disease onset can be from 11 months to 17 years [6]. Although the disease has been known for decades, a single tactic of its treatment has not yet been developed. In many respects, it depends on the variety of forms and their etiopathogenetic features. In particular, the main focus is on the use of drug therapy, and too little attention is paid to plasmapheresis. Therefore, the main objective of this study is to justify the need for plasmapheresis in the treatment of MG.

2. Etiology and pathogenesis

MG is a long-term neuromuscular disease that leads to various degrees of the skeletal muscles weakness. The most commonly affected muscles are those of the eyes, face, and swallowing [7]. In this case, IgG antibodies appear to nicotine acetylcholine (ACh) receptors of the postsynaptic membrane, which leads to the muscle weakness increase [8]. In some cases, antibodies can also emerge to the muscle-specific kinase (MuSK) [9]. In this case, antibodies against MuSK can produce plasmoblasts, and in such cases, removal of B-lymphocytes does not exclude recurrence of MG [10]. It also does not exclude autoantibodies presence to other postsynaptic proteins (anti-titin, anti-integrin antibodies) in small amounts [11–13].

3. Drug therapy

3.1 Cholinesterase inhibitors

Cholinesterase inhibitors (pyridostigmine bromide) delay the disease progression and increase the availability of ACh on the motor end membranes and lead to their strength increase [14]. Cholinergic side effects, including hyperactivation of the smooth muscles of the urinary bladder and intestines causing diarrhea, abdominal cramps, increased salivation, sweating, and bradycardia, are dose limiting and lead to noncompliance to the treatment plan [15].

3.2 Corticosteroids

The most common tactic for MG treatment is based on corticosteroids therapy [16]. However, such therapy is not deprived of a large number of adverse reactions. They lead to *Cushingoid syndrome*. Glucocorticoids, in particular, are *diabetogenic* hormones for they suppress glucose consumption by the tissues, and its production by the liver becomes increased. Besides, they can also directly suppress the release of insulin, thus showing that β-cells of pancreatic islets are one of their targets. Other complication of long glucocorticoid therapy is *osteoporosis*. It is considered that these hormones inhibit proliferation and differentiation of osteoblasts and stimulate their apoptosis. There is also an indirect mechanism of bones resorption caused by secondary hyperparathyreosis due to intestinal calcium adsorption decrease. Glucocorticoids effect on hypothalamus and gonads causes *hypogonadism* [17]. Development of chronic inflammatory polyneuropathy is also described [18]. There are evidences about correlation between such intensive and prolonged immunosuppressive therapy and the onset of tumors [19, 20].

3.3 Immunoglobulins

Administration of large doses of immunoglobulins does lead to such serious complications as aseptic meningitis, hemolytic anemia, cardiac rhythm disorders, and neurologic frustration in children with thrombotic thrombocytopenic purpura. Arthritis, thromboembolic complications, vasculitis, and a systemic lupus erythematosus are the side effects of autoantibodies and circulating immune complexes. Besides, there are other complications such as lethal hypersensitive (allergic) myocarditis and refractory heart failure, rash and skin itch, a leucopenia, a neutropenia, fever, etc. [21–24]. Presence of immune complexes may be the cause of it [25]; however, the main cause that must be recognized is the technology of immunoglobulins preparation from thousands (!) of donors having different blood types with full set of anti-A and anti-B isohemagglutinins (α and β), which lead to destruction of the corresponding erythrocytes [26]. At the same time, plasma exchange was necessary to relieve such hemolytic complication [27].

3.4 Rituximab

In the recent years, treatment of autoimmune diseases with rituximab—chimeric monoclonal antibody to CD20 antigen of B-lymphocytes—has become rather widespread, which should reduce the production of autoantibodies [28]. Rituximab is believed to be the first choice therapy [7]. Nevertheless, there are also complications of such treatment described leading even to *fulminant hepatitis* and *multiple organ failure* development [28–30]. Rituximab, cetuximab, and panitumumab have direct nephrotoxic effect [31]. *Rituximab* and *alemtuzumab* are reported to cause interstitial pneumonia development [32]. Prospectively, after rituximab treatment, neutropenia with pneumonia and other infectious complications may develop in up to 17% [33, 34]. There are reports about development of male infertility due to either gonadal dysfunction or antisperm autoantibodies production [35]. In addition, as noted above, removal of B-cells is not always accompanied by decrease in the autoantibodies reproduction [10].

4. Plasmapheresis

Considering the disease autoimmune nature, direct removal of antibodies by plasmapheresis is more effective [9, 36–38]. It causes normalization of immunoglobulin levels and reduction of the circulating immune complexes (CICs) in 1.7–2 times. The overall subjective improvement is observed in 94% of patients after a primary set of five plasma exchange procedures with their addition if necessary [39]. In severe cases, patients can be quickly disconnected from the artificial lung ventilation, but it is a relatively short-term effect and requires repeated sets of procedures [40].

Nevertheless, along with plasmapheresis, the same results are obtained by intensive intravenous immunoglobulin administration at a dose of 0.4 g/kg daily for 3 or 5 days [41, 42]. Though, using intensive plasmapheresis, we can achieve better results in the treatment of myasthenic crises, rather than by intravenous administration of immunoglobulins, the course of which costs $78.814 [43–47]. Immunoadsorption methods are also used; however, the best results are achieved in combination with plasma exchange [16].

It is advisable to carry out three to five procedures of plasmapheresis with removal of plasma up to 2.0–2.5 ml/kg of the body weight [48]. It is also possible to carry out daily procedures of plasma exchange removing smaller amounts of plasma, instead of the abovementioned plasma exchange, being carried out every other day [49]. Similarly, plasma exchange provides faster positive effect (already after the first procedure) in patients resistant to rituximab [50]. Nevertheless, carrying out plasma exchange along with rituximab treatment appeared more effective [51].

Plasmapheresis before thymectomy greatly facilitates the postoperative period [52–55]. Moreover, in cases when thymoma recurs postoperatively after a course of a plasma exchange, its involution is observed [56].

In juvenile forms of MG, plasmapheresis with immunoglobulins appears successful [57, 58], and it was noted that *plasma exchange yields more stable results* than IVIG therapy [44].

It should be noted that in the earliest symptoms of MG such as weakness of the cervical paraspinal muscles (*dropped head syndrome*), plasma exchange and immunoadsorption are justified [59].

The use of specific IgG-immunoadsorption to remove antibodies to ACh receptors [60] seems prospective as well as new systems for cascade plasmapheresis [53, 61].

At a cascade plasma exchange, the level of soluble molecules of intercellular adhesion decreases more effectively and the quantity of the T-regulating cells increases [62]. After a cascade plasma exchange, they observe increase in the $SatO_2$ levels associated with decrease in pCO_2 [63].

Nevertheless, in the comparable groups of patients with MG, there were no significant differences noted in the effectiveness of immunoadsorption or cascade plasmapheresis [64, 65]. On the other hand, there were no benefits found of immunoglobulin transfusions before cascade plasmapheresis or immunoadsorption [66]. After a cascade plasma exchange, they also noted a decrease in cytotoxic activity of the natural killer cells that even more improves the effectiveness of such treatment [67].

MG development is also possible in infants due to "graft-versus-host" disease (GVHD) following bone marrow transplantation. The course of plasmapheresis with subsequent administration of immunoglobulins was quite effective [68].

Our own experience shows that there are two possible applications of plasmapheresis. In myasthenic crises accompanied by swallowing and breathing disorders when patients need artificial lung ventilation, it is really necessary to urgently conduct a massive plasma exchange, removing 1–1.5 of the total plasma volume (TPV) with compensation with albumin and fresh frozen donor plasma for four to five procedures every day or every other day [69, 70]. The same tactic is described in the American Society for Apheresis Guidelines on the Use of Therapeutic Apheresis in Clinical Practice [71].

Then, to achieve a more stable remission, it is necessary to repeat procedures of less massive plasmapheresis at intervals of 2–4 weeks, removing only 0.3–0.5 TPV. The same tactic is used in less severe degrees of the disease, when the removed plasma volume can be compensated only by crystalloid solutions. In this case, the primary course also consists of four such plasmapheresis procedures, followed by one procedure every 1–2 months. Given the fact that MG can be observed in young children up to the development of myasthenic crises, it is desirable to use equipment with a small volume of filling. In our practice, we use a device for membrane plasmapheresis called "Hemophenix" ("Trackpore Technology," Russia) with an internal filling volume up to 70 ml, which can be used even in unstable hemodynamics, including in children. The advantage is a single-needle access using any peripheral vein.

Our practice includes 15 patients with MG. Two of them were in acute stage of the myasthenic crisis with respiratory failure, requiring connection to artificial lungs ventilation. One of them was a girl of 8 years old, who had complication of GVHD on the background of lymphocytic leukemia. She had already been on artificial lung ventilation for 10 days without visible effect (**Figure 1**). After two procedures of plasma exchange in a volume of 1.2 TPV, she was already able to breathe herself. In total, five such procedures were performed with a good effect of restoring the motor activity except for some left eyelid ptosis, which persisted after a month (**Figure 2**). The second patient had been on the artificial lung ventilation for 2 weeks in one of the clinics in Sofia, Bulgaria (**Figure 3**). Also, after two plasma exchange procedures, it was possible to switch him off the artificial lung ventilation (**Figure 4**), and after the last fourth procedure, he was already able to move without assistance and was discharged from the clinic.

The other patients were in different degrees of MG severity, and they performed a conventional plasmapheresis in the volume of 0.3–0.5 TPV with replacement of the removed plasma with an isotonic solution of sodium chloride. The course of treatment consisted of four such procedures, conducted every other day. Most of the procedures were performed in outpatient settings. The main task was to stabilize the condition and prevent the disease recurrence. One of them was in

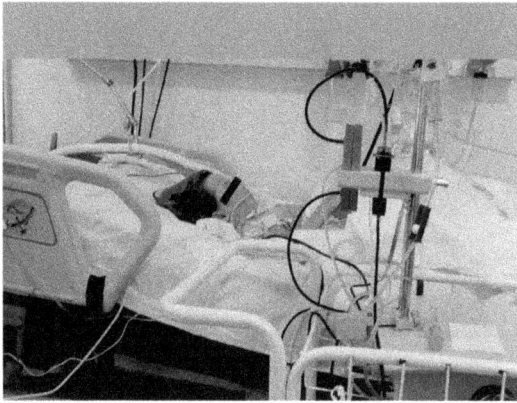

Figure 1.
Girl M of 8 years old and 18 kg body weight. Myasthenic crisis with artificial ventilation for 10 days. Plasma exchange using the "Hemophenix" device.

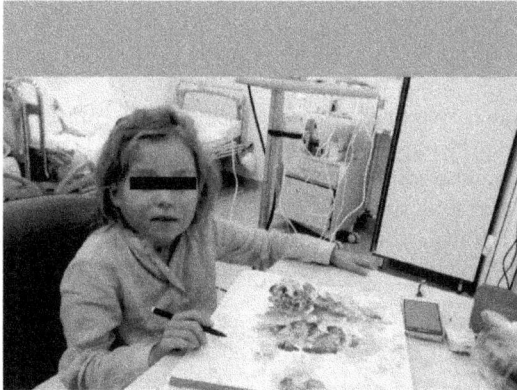

Figure 2.
The same girl a month after the course of plasma exchange.

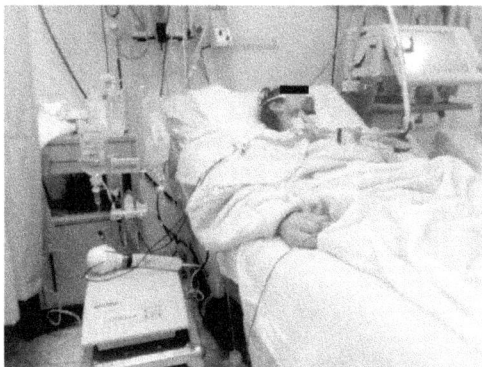

Figure 3.
Patient T of 28 years old. The first session of plasma exchange on the device "Hemophenix" on the background of artificial lung ventilation, carried out for 2 weeks.

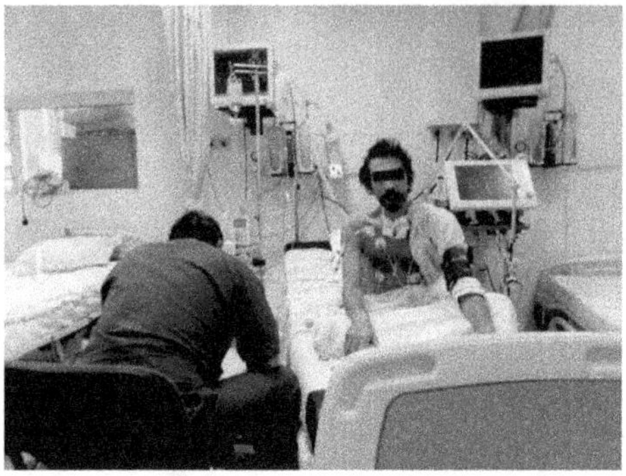

Figure 4.
The same patient after two sessions of plasma exchange. Disconnected from the ventilator.

quite serious condition and was able to move only with someone's assistance. After the primary course of plasmapheresis, we followed the tactics of a "programmed" plasmapheresis once per month, which enabled him to return to his physical work of an auto mechanic. The follow-up period is 6 years.

5. Conclusion

The autoimmune nature of the disease undoubtedly is an indication for plasmapheresis since it is the only way to remove large-molecule pathological products (autoantibodies, immune complexes) that cannot be excreted by the kidneys. Our experience shows that after such courses of plasmapheresis, conducted twice a year, it is possible to practically reduce the doses of corticosteroids and other medicines by half and, thereby, avoid the toxic consequences of their use.

Author details

Valerii Voinov
First I.P. Pavlov State Medical University of Saint Petersburg, Russia

*Address all correspondence to: voinof@mail.ru

IntechOpen

References

[1] Silvestri NJ, Wolfe GI. Myasthenia gravis. Seminars in Neurology. 2012;**32**(3):215-226

[2] Lin CW, Chen TC, Jou JR, Woung LC. Update on ocular myasthenia gravis in Taiwan. Taiwan Journal of Ophthalmology. 2018;**8**(2):67-73

[3] Al-Bassam W, Kubicki M, Bailey M, et al. Characteristics, incidence, and outcome of patients admitted to the intensive care unit with myasthenia gravis. Journal of Critical Care. 2018;**45**:90-94

[4] Martinka I, Fulova M, Spalekova M, Spalek P. Epidemiology of myasthenia gravis in Slovakia in the years 1977-2015. Neuroepidemiology. 2018;**50**(3-4):153-159

[5] Peragallo JH. Pediatric myasthenia gravis. Seminars in Pediatric Neurology. 2017;**24**(2):116-121

[6] Castro D, Derisavifard S, Anderson M, et al. Juvenile myasthenia gravis: A twenty-year experience. Journal of Clinical Neuromuscular Disease. 2013;**14**(3):95-102

[7] Stetefeld HR, Schroeter M. Myasthenic crisis. Fortschritte der Neurologie-Psychiatrie 2018;**86**(5):301-307(article in German)

[8] Nakamura R, Makino T, Hanada T, et al. Heterogeneity of auto-antibodies against nAChR in myasthenic serum and their pathogenic roles in experimental autoimmune myasthenia gravis. Journal of Neuroimmunology. 2018;**320**:64-75

[9] Yamada C, Teener JW, Robertson D, et al. Maintenance plasmapheresis treatment for muscle specific kinase antibody positive myasthenia gravis patients. Journal of Clinical Apheresis. 2014;**29**(1):37-38

[10] Stathopoulos P, Kumar A, Heiden JAV, et al. Mechanisms underlying B cell immune dysregulation and autoantibody production in MuSK myasthenia gravis. Annals of the New York Academy of Sciences. 2018;**1412**(1):154-165

[11] Misra MK, Damotte V, Hollenbach JA. The immunogenetics of neurological disease. Immunology. 2018;**153**(4):399-414

[12] Ruff RL, Lisak RP. Nature and action of antibodies in myasthenia gravis. Neurologic Clinics. 2018;**36**(2):275-291

[13] Yi JS, Guptil JT, Stathopoulos P, et al. B cells in the pathophysiology of myasthenia gravis. Muscle & Nerve. 2018;**57**(2):172-184

[14] Farrugia ME, Ckeary M, Carmichael C. A retrospective study of acetylcholine receptor antibody positive ocular myasthenia in the west of Scotland. Journal of the Neurological Sciences. 2017;**382**:84-86

[15] Petrov KA, Kharlamova AD, Lenina OA, et al. Specific inhibition of acetylcholinesterase as an approach to decrease muscarinic side effects during myasthenia gravis treatment. Scientific Reports. 2018;**8**(1):304

[16] Schneider-Gold C, Krenzer M, Klinker E, et al. Immunoadsorption versus plasma exchange versus combination for treatment of myasthenic deterioration. Therapeutic Advances in Neurological Disorders. 2016;**9**(4):297-303

[17] Compston JE. Management of bone disease in patients on long term glucocorticoid therapy. Gut. 1999;**44**(6):770-772

[18] Chroni E, Veltsista D, Gavanozi E, et al. Pure sensory chronic

inflammatory polyneuropathy: Rapid deterioration after steroid treatment. BMC Neurology. 2015;**15**:27

[19] Pasquet F, Pavic M, Ninet J, Hot A. Autoimmune diseases and cancers. Part I: Cancers complicating autoimmune diseases and their treatment. Rev Mad Interne (French). 2014;**35**(5):310-316

[20] Giat E, Ehrenfeld M, Shoenfeld Y. Cancer and autoimmune diseases. Autoimmunity Reviews. 2017;**16**(10):1049-1057

[21] Lorenzana A, Armin S, Sharma A, et al. Cerebral infarctions after intravenous immunoglobulin therapy for ITR in child. Pediatric Neurology. 2014;**50**(2):188-191

[22] Bharath V, Eckert K, Kang M, et al. Incidence and natural history of intravenous immunoglobulin-induced aseptic meningitis: A retrospective review at a single tertiary care center. Transfusion. 2015;**55**(11):2597-2605

[23] Charhon N, Bonnet A, Schmitt Z, Charpiat B. A case of circulatory collapse during intravenous immunoglobulin therapy: A manageable adverse effect! Anaesthesia Critical Care & Pain Medicine. 2015;**34**(2):113-114

[24] Thornby KA, Henneman A, Brown DA. Evidence-based strategies to reduce intravenous immunoglobulin-induced headaches. The Annals of Pharmacotherapy. 2015;**49**(6):715-726

[25] Zimring JC. Do immune complexes play a role in hemolytic sequelae of intravenous immune globuilin? Transfusion. 2015;**55**(Suppl. 2):S86-S89

[26] Branch DR. Anti-A and anti-B: What are they and where do they come from? Transfusion. 2015;**55**(Suppl. 2):S74-S79

[27] Welsh KJ, Bai Y. Therapeutic plasma exchange as a therapeutic modality for the treatment of IVIG complications. Journal of Clinical Apheresis. 2015;**30**(6):371-374

[28] Ruch J, McMahon B, Ramsey G, Kwaan HC. Catastrophic multiple organ ischemia due to an anti-Pr cold agglutinin developing in a patient with mixed cryoglobulinemia after treatment with rituximab. American Journal of Hematology. 2009;**84**(2):120-122

[29] Sagnelli E, Pisaturo M, Sagnelli C, Coppola N. Rituximab-based treatment, HCV replication, and hepatic flares. Clinical & Developmental Immunology. 2012;**2012**:945950

[30] Yazici O, Sendur MA, Aksoy S. Hepatitis C virus reactivation in cancer patients in the era of targeted therapies. World Journal of Gastroenterology. 2014;**20**(22):6716-6724

[31] Abbas A, Mitza MM, Ganti AK, Tendulkar K. Renal toxicities of targeted therapies. Targeted Oncology. 2015;**10**(4):487-499

[32] Barber NA, Ganti AK. Pulmonary toxicities from targeted therapies: A review. Targeted Oncology. 2011;**6**(4):235-243

[33] Deborska-Materkowska D, Kozińska-Przybyl O, Mikaszewska-Sokolewicz M, Durlik M. Fatal late-onset pneumocystis pneumonia after rituximab: Administration for posttransplantation recurrence of focal segmental glomerulosclerosis-case report. Transplantation Proceedings. 2014;**46**(8): 2908-2911

[34] Lentine KL, Axelrod D, Klein C, et al. Early clinical complications after ABO-incompatible live-donor kidney transplantation: A national study of Medicare-insured recipients. Transplantation. 2014;**98**(1):54-65

[35] Tiseo BC, Cocuzza M, Bonfa F, et al. Male fertility potential alteration in rheumatic diseases: A systematic review. International Braz J Urol. 2016;42(1):11-21

[36] Dasararaju R, Man S, Marques M, Williams L. Seasonal variations in myasthenia gravis patients requiring therapeutic plasma exchange. Journal of Clinical Apheresis. 2014;29(1):36

[37] Lánez-Andrés JM, Gascón-Giménez F, Coret-Ferrer F, et al. Therapeutic plasma exchange: Applications in neurology. Revista de Neurologia. 2015;60(3):120-131

[38] Gotterer L, Li Y. Maintenance immunosuppression in myasthenia gravis. Journal of the Neurological Sciences. 2016;369:294-302

[39] Yamada C, Pham HP, Wu Y, et al. Report of the ASFA apheresis registry on muscle specific kinase antibody positive myasthenia gravis. Journal of Clinical Apheresis. 2016;32(1):5-11

[40] Kosachev VD, Yulev NM, Bechik SL. Plasma exchange for complex treating of myasthenia. Efferent Therapy. 2006;12(2):28-31 (Rus)

[41] Barth D, Nabavi N, Ng E, et al. Comparison of IVIg and PLEX in patients with myasthenia gravis. Neurology. 2011;76:2017-2023

[42] Ortiz-Salas P, Velez-Van-Meerbeke A, Galvis-Gomez CA, Rodriguez QJH. Human immunoglobulin versus plasmapheresis in Guillain-Barré syndrome and myasthenia gravis: A meta-analysis. Journal of Clinical Neuromuscular Disease. 2016;18(1):1-11

[43] Hellmann MA, Mosberg-Galili R, Lotan I, Steiner I. Maintenance IVIg therapy in myasthenia gravis does not affect disease activity. Journal of the Neurological Sciences. 2014;338:39-42

[44] Liew WK, Powell CA, Sloan SR, et al. Comparison of plasmapheresis and intravenous immunoglobulin as maintenance therapy for juvenile myasthenia gravis. JAMA Neurology. 2014;71(5):575-580

[45] Morgan SM, Shaz BH, Pavenski K, et al. The top clinical trial opportunities in therapeutic apheresis and neurology. Journal of Clinical Apheresis. 2014;29(6):331-335

[46] Dhawan PS, Goodman BP, Harper CM, et al. IVIG versus PLEX in the treatment of worsening myasthenia gravis: What is the evidence?: A critically appraised topic. The Neurologist. 2015;19(5):145-148

[47] Furlan JC, Barth D, Barnett C, Bril V. Cost-minimization analysis comparing intravenous immunoglobulin with plasma exchange in the management of patients with myasthenia gravis. Muscle & Nerve. 2015;53(6):872-876

[48] Köhler W, Bucka C, Klingel R. A randomized and controlled study comparing immunoadsorption and plasma exchange in myasthenic crisis. Journal of Clinical Apheresis. 2011;26(6):347-355

[49] Trikha I, Singh S, Goyal V, et al. Comparative efficacy of low dose, daily versus alternative day plasma exchange in severe myasthenia gravis: A randomized trial. Journal of Neurology. 2007;254:989-995

[50] Nowak RJ. Response of patients with refractory myasthenia gravis to rituximab: A retrospective study. Therapeutic Advances in Neurological Disorders. 2011;4(5):259-266

[51] Hayashi R, Tahara M, Oeda T, et al. A case of refractory generalized myasthenia gravis with anti-acetylcholine receptor antibodies

treated with rituximab. Rinshō
Shinkeigaku. 2015;55(4):227-232
(Japan)

[52] Gold R, Schneider-Gold C. Current
and future standard in treatment of
myasthenia gravis. Neurotherapeutics.
2008;5(4):535-541

[53] Konishi T. Plasmapheresis in
patients with myasthenia gravis. Nippon
Rinsho. 2008;66(6):1165-1171 (Japan)

[54] El-Bawab H, Hajjar W, Rafay
M, et al. Plasmapheresis before
thymectomy in myasthenia gravis:
Routine versus selective protocols.
European Journal of Cardiovascular
Surgery. 2009;35(3):392-397

[55] Yeh JH, Chen WH, Huang KM, Chiu
HC. Prethymectomy plasmapheresis in
myasthenia gravis. Journal of Clinical
Apheresis. 2005;20(4):217-221

[56] Jiang W, Yu Q. Case report of
thymoma tumor reduction following
plasmapheresis. Medicine (Baltimore).
2015;94(47):e2173

[57] Rybojad B, Lesiuk W, Fialkowska A,
et al. Management of myasthenic crisis
in a child. Anaesthesiology Intensive
Therapy. 2013;45(2):82-84

[58] Kroczka S, Stasiak K, Kaciński
M. Neurophysiological parameters
in myasthenia gravis in children in
diagnostic and therapeutic view.
Przegląd Lekarski. 2016;73(3):119-123

[59] Tamai M, Hashimoto T, Isobe
T, et al. Treatment of myasthenia
gravis with dropped head: A
report of 2 cases and review of the
literature. Neuromuscular Disorders.
2015;25(5):429-431

[60] Zisimopoulou P, Lagoumintzis G,
Kostelidou K, et al. Towards antigen-
specific apheresis of pathogenic
autoantibodies as a further step
in the treatment of myasthenia

gravis by plasmapheresis. Journal of
Neuroimmunology. 2008;15:95-103

[61] Batocchi AP, Evoli A, Di Schino
C, Tonali P. Therapeutic apheresis
in myasthenia gravis. Therapeutic
Apheresis. 2000;4(4):275-279

[62] Zhang L, Liu J, Wang H, et al.
Double filtration plasmapheresis
benefits myasthenia gravis patients
through an immunomodulatory action.
Journal of Clinical Neuroscience.
2014;21(9):1570-1574

[63] Yeh JH, Lin CM, Cheh WH,
Chiu HC. Effects of double filtration
plasmapheresis on nocturnal respiratory
function in myasthenic patients.
Artificial Organs. 2013;37(12):1076-1079

[64] Yeh JH, Chiu HC. Comparison
between double-filtration
plasmapheresis and immunoadsorption
plasmapheresis in the treatment
of patients with myasthenia
gravis. Journal of Neurology.
2000;247(7):510-513

[65] Pittayanon R, Treepraertsuk S,
Phanthumchinda K. Plasmapheresis
or intravenous immunoglobulin
for myasthenia gravis crisis in King
Chulalongkorn Memorial Hospital.
Journal of the Medical Association of
Thailand. 2009;92(4):478-482

[66] Liu JF, Wang WX, Xue J, et al.
Comparing the autoantibody levels
and clinical efficacy of double
plasmapheresis, immunoadsorption,
and intravenous immunoglobulin
for the treatment of late-onset
myasthenia gravis. Therapeutic
Apheresis and Dialysis.
2010;14(2):153-160

[67] Chien PJ, Yeh JH, Chiu HC, et al.
Inhibition of peripheral blood natural
killer cell cytotoxicity in patients
with myasthenia gravis treated with
plasmapheresis. European Journal of
Neurology. 2011;18(11):1350-1357

[68] Nakashima J, Itonaga H, Fujioka M, et al. Durable remission attained with plasmapheresis and intravenous immunoglobulin therapy in a patient with acute exacerbation of GVHD-related myasthenia gravis. Rinshō Ketsueki. 2018;**59**(5):480-484

[69] Voinov VA. Therapeutic Apheresis. Constanţa: Celebris; 2016. 403 p (Romania)

[70] Voinov VA, Kenarov PD. The Plasmapheresis as Intensive Treatment of Neurologic Diseases. St Petersburg: RITC FSPbGMU; 2018. p. 49

[71] Schwartz J, Padmanabhan A, Aqui N, et al. Guidelines on the use of therapeutic apheresis in clinical practice—Evidence-based approach from the writing committee of the American Society for Apheresis: The sixth special issue. Journal of Clinical Apheresis. 2016;**28**:149-338

Chapter 6

Anticholinesterases

Zeynep Özdemir and Mehmet Abdullah Alagöz

Abstract

Acetylcholinesterase (AChE) and butyrylcholinesterase (BChE) are known serine hydrolase enzymes responsible for the hydrolysis of acetylcholine (ACh). Although the role of AChE in cholinergic transmission is well known, the role of BChE has not been elucidated sufficiently. The hydrolysis of acetylcholine in the synaptic healthy brain cells is mainly carried out by AChE; it is accepted that the contribution to the hydrolysis of BChE is very low, but both AChE and BChE are known to play an active role in neuronal development and cholinergic transmission. Myasthenia gravis (MG) is a muscle disease characterized by weakness in skeletal muscles and rapid fatigue. Anticholinesterases, which are not only related to the immune origin of the disease but also have only symptomatic benefit, have an indispensable role in the treatment of MG. Pyridostigmine, distigmine, neostigmine, and ambenonium are the standard anticholinesterase drugs used in the symptomatic treatment of MG. All of these compounds may increase the response of the myasthenic muscle to recurrent nerve impulses, primarily by protecting the endogenous ACh.

Keywords: acetylcholine, acetylcholinesterase, butyrylcholinesterase, anticholinesterases, neostigmine, pyridostigmine, distigmine, ambenonium, myasthenia gravis

1. Introduction

The autonomic nervous system (ANS) works out of our request, and it differs from the somatic system with this feature. Autonomic afferent and efferent fibers enter and exit the central nervous system through the spinal and cranial nerves. It connects with the medulla spinalis and intermediate neurons, which mediate autonomic reflexes in the brain stem [1, 2]. Changes in the internal and external environment and emotional factors affect autonomic activity through fibers, which descend from the hypothalamus. ANS shows its effect through neuromediators. Acetylcholine (ACh) and noradrenaline (NA) are the main neurotransmitters in the autonomic nervous system. ACh is released from all preganglionic endings. ACh is secreted from all postganglionic parasympathetic fibers, and it acts through muscarinic receptors [3, 4]. Autonomic nervous system disorders may occur with an abnormally high parasympathetic activity or abnormally low parasympathetic activity and/or abnormally high sympathetic activity or abnormally low sympathetic activity. MG, a neuromuscular junction disease that occurs due to ACh receptor deficiency in the postsynaptic membrane at the neuromuscular junction, is one of these disorders. The origin of the disease is thymus, because myoid cells form the source of receptor antigens. ACh release in the normal muscular junction leads to a localized end-plate potential, resulting in muscle contraction [5]. Although MG patients have normal nerve anatomy and function, there is a decrease in the number of postsynaptic ACh receptors. During a muscle contraction under normal conditions, the release of ACh, which is caused by impulses along the axon, decreases gradually in each impulse. This decrease does not cause problems in the postsynaptic membrane when there is no pathology. However, in addition to the reduced number of receptors in MG, the ACh-receptor complex is also decreasing gradually; therefore, rapid fatigue is observed [6, 7].

2. Acetylcholine and cholinergic receptors

The neurotransmitter is ACh in all of the preganglionic autonomic fibers constituting the peripheral parts of the autonomic nervous system, in all postganglionic parasympathetic fibers and in several postganglionic sympathetic nerve fibers, and these ACh release fibers are called cholinergic fibers [8]. ACh is synthesized in the cytosol at the end of the nerve fibers, and then it is transported into the vesicles from the membrane of the vesicles (**Figure 1**). ACh is stored here in a very dense manner, with about 10,000 molecules in each vesicle. When an action potential reaches the nerve end, a large number of calcium channels are opened on the nerve end, since it has a large number of voltage-gated calcium channels.

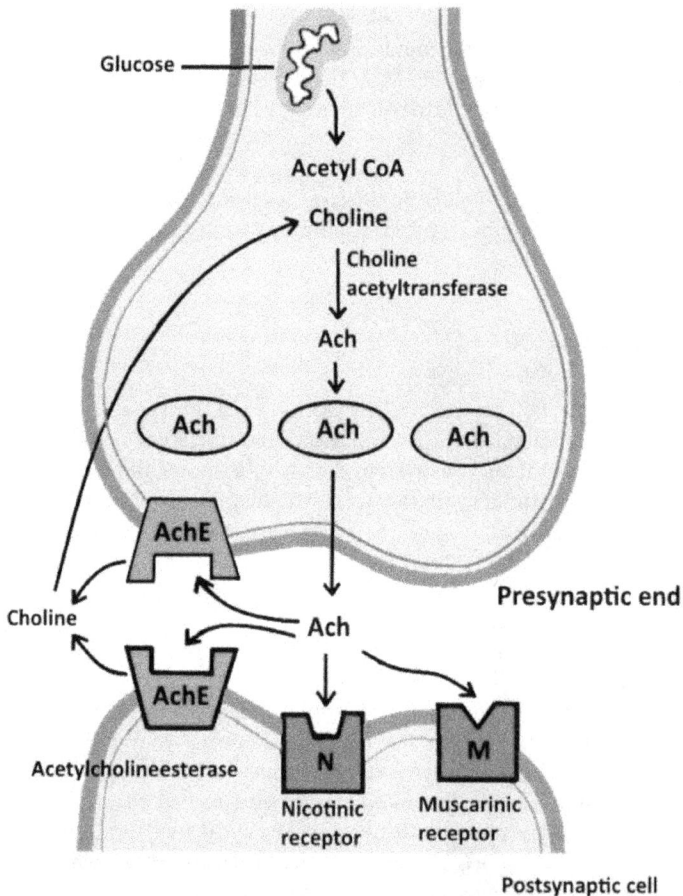

Figure 1.
Biosynthesis, transmission, and inactivation of ACh [3].

As a result, the calcium concentration in the nerve end increases by 100 times; this increases the speed of incorporation of ACh vesicles with the nerve end membrane by 10,000 times. This incorporation allows the exocytosis of acetylcholine to the synaptic range by causing rupture of many vesicles. About 125 vesicles are usually ruptured with each action potential. The ACh is then broken up with AChE in a few milliseconds to the acetate ion and choline. Choline is taken back to the nerve end to be used in the formation of ACh again [9].

Studies have shown that many tissues respond to stimulation and inhibition are generated by compounds, which mimic the action of neuronal release of ACh or the neurotransmitter administered externally. Peripheral cholinergic receptors interacting with ACh are found in the parasympathetic postganglionic nerve endings in the smooth muscles and neuromuscular junction in the skeletal muscles. Cholinergic receptors are divided into two groups, namely nicotinic and muscarinic. The distribution of muscarinic receptors in the brain adapts to the distribution of ACh [10]. Receptors are mostly found in the striatum, neocortex, hippocampus, superior colliculus, locus coeruleus, and pons nuclei; whereas, the quantity of them in the hypothalamus, spinal cord, and cortex is low. These receptors in neuromuscular motor ends and ganglia are the first neurotransmitter receptors that have been isolated and purified in active form. It is contemplated that the receptor is comprised of two polypeptide chain monomers, which are connected to each other by a disulfide bond and have five subunits. When ACh is bound to these receptors, it allows the passage of the small cations such as Ca^{++}, Na^+, and K^+ by leading to an increase in membrane permeability. The physiological effect of this condition is the formation of depolarization at the motor ends and consequently the muscular contraction or the continuation of nerve stimulation at the neuromuscular junction. Muscarinic receptors play an important role in regulating the functions of organs stimulated by the autonomic nervous system. The effect of ACh on these receptors in parasympathetic synapses may be stimulating or inhibiting. ACh both stimulates the secretion by activating the salivary glands and leads to the contraction of the respiratory system. The compound also inhibits cardiac contractions and relaxes the smooth muscles in the blood vessels. Recent studies have shown that there are five subtypes of muscarinic receptors (M_1, M_2, M_3, M_4, and M_5). M_1 is found in neuronal structures such as the central nervous system and ganglions, M_2 is found in the heart, M_3 is found in the smooth muscles in the glands, and M_4 is also found in the striatum and lungs [8–10].

2.1 Cholinesterase enzymes and cholinesterase inhibitors

AChE is a hydrolytic enzyme of the class of the serine hydrolase enzyme, which plays a major role in the hydrolysis of ACh in cholinergic synapses of the autonomic nervous system and central nervous system [11]. Electron microscopy studies using histochemical techniques have shown that this enzyme is located on both the nerve endings and the postjunction or postsynaptic membrane at the cholinergic synapses or junctions. This enzyme, which is also called main cholinesterase, hydrolyzes ACh most rapidly among choline esters. It can also hydrolyze methacholine, but it is ineffective against benzoylcholine. A second type of cholinesterase, which is called pseudocholinesterase, breaks down acetylcholine more slowly. Because this enzyme is the most rapidly broken choline ester butyrylcholine, pseudocholinesterase is called butyrylcholinesterase (BChE). Butyrylcholinesterase is not found in synapses and does not contribute to the hydrolysis of acetylcholine [12]. Both AChE and BChE are polymorphic and exist as homomeric and heteromeric molecular forms characterized by subunit relationships and hydrodynamic properties. Heteromeric molecular forms contain catalytic subunits linked to the lipid or triple helix collagen tail and are often referred to as asymmetric or A forms of AChE. The G_1, G_2, and G_4 forms, which are homomeric hydrophilic globular forms of AChE, contain one, two, and four identical subunits, respectively. The G_4 form is secreted by neurons and secretory cells. An amphiphilic glycophospholipid-bound form is a dimer of G_2, which has two subunits having a glycophospholipid link to the cell membrane. Less polymorphism is observed in BChE, and only hydrophilic and asymmetric forms have been defined for this enzyme [11].

The structure of AChE reveals an active site containing a catalytic triad-glutamate (E327), histidine (H440), and serine (S200) at the base of a narrow valley about 20 A depth. This general amino acid arrangement represents the serine hydrolase enzyme family. The gorge in AChE is coated with 14 aromatic amino acids consisting of phenylalanine, tyrosine or tryptophan, and the base of the gorge contains a number of anionic residues, which are collectively responsible for the interaction of ACh with the positively charged trimethylammonium group and the acceleration of binding of the cationic ligands. BChE contains six less aromatic amino acids than AChE in the gorge. These structural studies help to elucidate the molecular basis of the specificity between the active center and the ligand. In particular, the main substrate differences between AChE and BChE can be determined by the presence of two phenylalanines (F288 and F290), providing a rigid acyl binding pocket in AChE. In addition, replacement of these amino acids with leucine and valine to provide a less structurally restricted pocket in BChE can also determine the main substrate differences between AChE and BChE. In addition, AChE contains a peripheral anionic region responsible for allosteric inhibition by cationic ligand interactions in the catalytic region. This peripheral anionic region proposed by Changeux in 1966 links agents such as propidium to residues around the edge of the gorge. This peripheral anionic region may play a role in the catalytic process by mediating substrate inhibition [13–17].

The effects of ACh released from autonomic and somatic motor nerves are terminated by enzymatic degradation of the molecule by AChE that is present in high concentrations in cholinergic synapses and synthesized in both nerve and muscle tissues [18]. The drugs, which inhibit AChE, are called anticholinesterase agents. The characteristic pharmacological effects of anticholinesterases occur primarily by inhibiting the hydrolysis of AChE by the AChE enzyme in cholinergic pathways. Inhibition of cholinesterases induces ACh receptors by leading increased ACh in nerve synapses and neuromuscular junction. Continuous stimulation of ACh receptors results in cholinergic synaptic paralysis and central and peripheral clinical symptoms in the central nervous system, autonomic ganglia, parasympathetic and sympathetic nerve endings, and somatic nerves due to the accumulation of ACh in the motor end plates. Muscarinic effects due to parasympathetic activity and nicotinic effects due to sympathetic activity are seen. The main symptoms and signs depend on the balance between muscarinic and nicotinic receptors [8, 18].

Inhibition of the AChE prolongs the life of the neurotransmitter at the junction, thus resulting in pharmacological effects similar to those observed when acetylcholine is administered. AChE is the primary target of these drugs, but BChE is also inhibited. Anti-AChEs are used in the treatment of diseases such as myasthenia gravis, atony in the gastrointestinal tract, glaucoma, and Alzheimer's disease. These compounds are also used as nerve gases and insecticides. Anti-AChE agents can be divided into three groups based on their mechanism of action: competitive agonists, short-acting inhibitors, and long-acting inhibitors [19]. Before World War II, only reversible anti-ChE agents were known and their prototype is physostigmine. Organophosphates as highly toxic chemicals, which were first developed as agricultural insecticides, were also developed as a potential chemical warfare agent shortly before World War II. It is known that the excessive toxicity of these compounds is due to the irreversible inactivation of AChE. Thus, organophosphate inhibitors are sometimes referred to as "irreversible cholinesterase inhibitors." Strong nucleophiles such as pralidoxime can break phosphorus enzyme binding [9, 19].

Anti-AChEs, which are currently used for treatment in the postoperative period of intestinal system and atony of the smooth muscles of bladder, glaucoma, myasthenia gravis, and termination of the effects of competitive neuromuscular muscle relaxants produce nonselectively both muscarinic and nicotinic effects as indirect effects by increasing the ACh concentration. Long-acting and hydrophobic ChE inhibitors are also the only inhibitors with limited, well-documented efficacy in the treatment of dementia symptoms of Alzheimer's disease [8, 20].

MG is a muscle disease characterized by weakness in skeletal muscles and rapid fatigue. Anti-AChEs, which are not only related to the immune origin of the disease but have only symptomatic benefit, have an indispensable role in the treatment of MG. Pyridostigmine, distigmin, neostigmine, and ambenonium are the standard anticholinesterase drugs used in the symptomatic treatment of MG. All of these compounds may increase the response of the myasthenic muscle to recurrent nerve impulses, primarily by protecting the endogenous ACh [8, 21, 22].

2.1.1 Pyridostigmine

The most commonly used anti-ChE in daily treatment is pyridostigmine bromide (**Figure 2**). The effect of the drug starts in 15–30 min, reaches maximum in 1–2 hours, and lasts 3–4 hours or longer. Pyridostigmine bromide, used for the treatment of MG and for protection against exposure to nerve agents, is a carbamate-derived reversible AChE inhibitor [23–25]. Due to the quaternary amine structure, it is relatively weakly absorbed from the gastrointestinal system. The elimination of half-life of pyridostigmine bromide after a single dose of 60 mg in healthy volunteers was found to be 200 min. This requires frequent usage. Ninety-nine percent of AChE inhibitors, including pyridostigmine bromide, are administered orally [26–28].

2.1.2 Distigmine

Distigmine is a carbamate-derived reversible ChE inhibitor. The compound synthesized chemically by Schmid has a chemical structure consisting of two molecules of pyridostigmine bonded together by hexamethylene bonds (**Figure 3**). Distigmine is clinically used in some Asian and European countries, including Japan and Germany, and the main clinical indication for distigmine is myasthenia gravis.

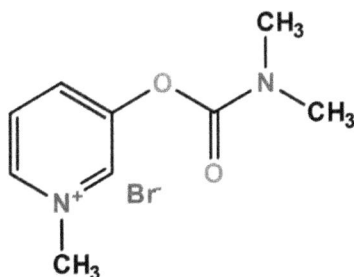

Figure 2.
Structure of pyridostigmine bromide.

However, in Japan, distigmin was also used for glaucoma and underactive bladder [29, 30].

2.1.3 Neostigmine

Neostigmine (**Figure 4**) is commonly used to reverse nondepolarizing neuromuscular blocking agents. The drug increases the rate of recovery from moderate nondepolarizing neuromuscular blockade and reduces the incidence of residual blockade. However, doses of neostigmine used in clinical practice may cause muscle weakness when administered after complete recovery from neuromuscular blockade. Since the first studies investigating the effects of neostigmine were performed in anesthetized patients, the results may be mixed with the presence of anesthetic agents, which are known to be in the neuromuscular blockade. Later, the effect of neostigmine was supported by the studies that the volunteers did not receive anesthetic agents. However, the effects of neostigmine on maximum voluntary muscle strength have not been previously investigated [31, 32].

2.1.4 Ambenonium

In addition, compounds, which are structurally different from the above-mentioned carbamates for the treatment of MG, are also used. One of them, bisquaternary inhibitor ambenonium dichloride (**Figure 5**), is known to be one of the compounds with the highest inhibition ability against AChE in sub-nM range [33].

The superior effect potential is unique for the compound, which does not form any covalent bonds with the active site of the enzyme. Binding studies on the AChE-ambenonium complex have shown that the compound is capable of making very

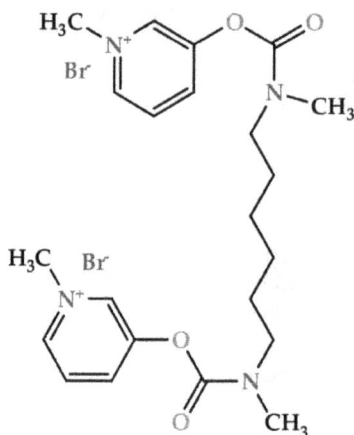

Figure 3.
Structure of distigmine.

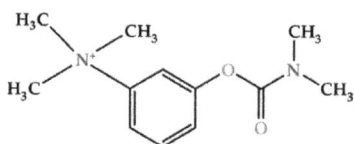

Figure 4.
Structure of neostigmine.

convenient contacts with the amino acids of the catalytic and peripheral AChE sites. Ambenonium produces less muscarinic side effects than carbamates. Unlike short-acting anti-AChE compounds, it is advantageous because it produces a larger and longer-lasting therapeutic effect during the night and waking period. In addition, the bisquaternary structure inhibits the passage from blood-brain barrier (BBB) after a conventional oral or intravenous route of administration. Another anti-AChE compound, edrophonium chloride (**Figure 6**), is used as a diagnostic tool for MG. It has a rapid onset and short pharmacological effect, so it cannot be used for therapeutic purposes [33, 34].

The optimal single oral dose of the anti-ChE agents can be determined empirically, when the MG is diagnosed. Basic records are made for a range of signs and symptoms, which reflect comprehension strength, vital capacity, and the strength of various muscle groups. The patient is given an oral dose of pyridostigmine at 30–60 mg, neostigmine at 7.5–15 mg, or ambenonium at 2.5–5 mg. Improvement in muscle strength and changes in other symptoms are recorded at frequent intervals until they return to the baseline state. After a baseline hour or longer, the drug is reintroduced, the dose is increased to one and a half times the initial amount, and the same observations are repeated. These repeats continue with increments of half the initial dose until the optimal dose is achieved. The duration of action between the oral doses is required to maintain the muscle strength of these drugs, which is usually 2–4 h for neostigmine, 3–6 h for pyridostigmine, or 3–8 h for ambenonium. However, the required dose may vary from day to day. Physical or emotional stress, intercurrent infections, and menstruation usually require an increase in the frequency or size of the dose. Unpredictable exacerbations and remissions of the myasthenic condition may require adjustment of the dosage. Pyridostigmine has sustained release tablets containing a total of 180 mg, 60 mg of this is released immediately and the drug concentration is 120 mg for several hours. This preparation is valuable in maintaining patients in periods of 6–8 h, but it should be limited to use before bedtime [5, 8, 35].

There is always a risk of cholinergic crisis, if the effects of anti-ChE drugs are weak and there is no any improvement in the symptoms of the disease even with high doses of AChE. In cholinergic crisis, nausea, vomiting, sweating, salivation, colic, diarrhea, miosis, bradycardia, etc., are observed and myasthenic weakness increases [7]. In addition, many drugs, including curariform agents,

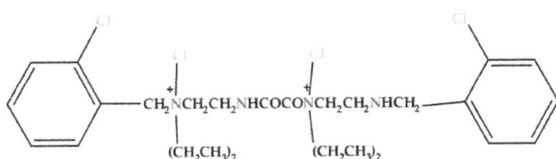

Figure 5.
Structure of ambenonium.

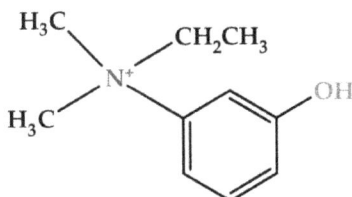

Figure 6.
Structure of edrophonium.

certain antibiotics, and general anesthetics prevent neuromuscular transmission. Therefore, the application of these drugs to patients with MG requires an appropriate adjustment of the anti-ChE dose and other measures [8].

2.2 Newly developed cholinesterase inhibitors for MG

Muscarinic cardiovascular and gastrointestinal side effects of anti-ChE agents can usually be controlled by atropine or other anticholinergic drugs. However, these anticholinergic drugs mask many side effects of an excessive amount of anti-ChE agents. Tolerance in most patients may eventually lead to muscarinic effects [5, 7, 35, 36]. For these reasons, it is aimed to investigate more effective drugs for the treatment of MG and to prevent the hepatotoxicity and known gastrointestinal side effects, while creating the targeted pharmacological effect with the synthetic analogues at the development stage.

Musilek et al. performed the synthesis of 20 new bis-isoquinolinium inhibitors (**Figure** 7) in a study and determined whether the compounds would be effective in the treatment of MG. They evaluated the newly prepared compounds *in vitro* on human recombinant AChE and human plasmatic BChE and compared the inhibitory capabilities of the compounds expressed as IC_{50} with ambenonium dichloride, edrophonium chloride, BW284c51, and ethopropazine hydrochloride, which have been selected as standard. In three of the compounds they have obtained, they had promising results in which their compounds inhibited both enzymes better than or similar to edrophonium and BW284c51, however, worse than ambenonium *in vitro*. The kinetic assays are confirmed noncompetitive inhibition of human-recombinant AChE (hAChE) with two promising new compounds selected [37].

In a study in which neostigmine, pyridostigmine, and physostigmine quaternary phenylcarbamates were synthesized and evaluated their activity, N-monophenylcarbamate analogues together with their precursors of neostigmine methyl sulfate and pyridostigmine bromide and the N-methylammonium analogues of phenserine, tolserine, cymserine, and phenylethylcymserine were synthesized as long-acting peripheral inhibitors of AChE or BChE (**Figure 8**). According to the results of the study, only N-phenylcarbamate of 3-dimethylamiophenol to N-phenylcarbamate of 3-hydroxy-1-methylpyridinium bromide compounds had marginal ChE inhibitor of activity and compound N(1)-methylammonium bromide of (−)-phenserine, (−)-tolserine, (−)-cymserine, and (−)-phenylethylcymserine were strong anti-ChEs [38].

Monarsen (EN101) is an antisense oligodeoxynucleotide, which acts at the level of mRNA and selectively reduces the production of тне enzymatic isoform of readthrough AChE (AChE-R) by the destruction of the AChE-R mRNA. This compound selectively lowers the AChE-R levels in both blood and muscle, but, does not affect the synaptic variant of synaptic AChE (AChE-S). It was tested in experimental

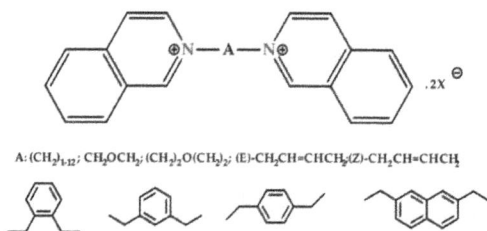

Figure 7.
Structure of bis-isoquinolinium derivatives.

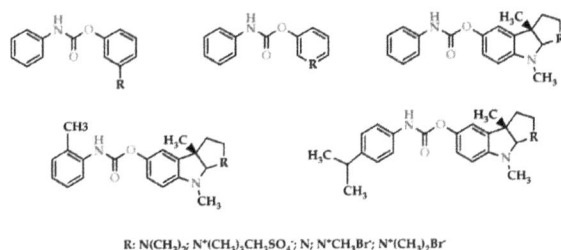

R: N(CH₃)₂; N⁺(CH₃)₃CH₃SO₄⁻; N; N⁺CH₃Br⁻; N⁺(CH₃)₂Br⁻

Figure 8.
Structure of neostigmine N-phenylcarbamate of 3-dimethylamiophenol and 3-hydroxy-1-methylpyridinium and N(1)-methylammonium bromide of (-)-phenserine, (-)-tolserine, (-)-cymserine, and (-)-phenylethylcymserine.

autoimmune MG rats that oral or intravenous administration of EN101 reduced AChE in blood and muscle and increased survival, muscle strength, and disease severity. The stabilization of the reduction of the compound motor action potential (CMAP) on the responsive neurostimulation system and muscles was also observed during the entire treatment. This effect has been found to be comparable to that of pyridostigmine, which is worn out for hours and causes significant fluctuations in muscle strength. It was also found that clinical and electrophysiological improvement was associated with a decrease in autoimmune responses [39–41].

3. Conclusions

Anti-ChEs have an indispensable role in the symptomatic treatment of the MG, which is not directed against the immune origin. AChE inhibitors improve neuromuscular conduction by preventing disruption of circulating ACh in the neuromuscular junction. The compounds used in the treatment of MG have a positive charge in the molecule to provide the peripheral effect of the action and minimal blood-brain barrier penetration. However, the most prescribed carbamate inhibitors may cause many serious side effects, such as carbamylation of AChE. As a result, it is important to individually arrange treatment for each MG patient. The effect of treatment should be optimized for vital muscles such as respiratory and swallowing; because, different muscles are affected by varying levels. Since the nonselective AChE inhibitors are the most effective compounds at the beginning of MG, the dosage of AChE inhibitors is ideally reduced as they develop strength by immunosuppressive therapy. Decrease in activity over time may be related to increased levels of the AChE-R isoform, which may cause morphological and physiological abnormalities in the neuromuscular junction. Myasthenia gravis (MG) is usually caused by antibodies either to the acetylcholine receptor (AChR) or to the muscle-specific tyrosine kinase (MuSK) or at the neuromuscular junction. Patients with MuSK antibodies generally do not respond to the treatment; whereas, patients with AChR antibodies respond specifically to the treatment. For these reasons, EN101, a selective AChE inhibitor that specifically targets the isoform of AChE (AChE-R), has been developed recently and the AChR-antibody may be important for symptomatic relief in seropositive MG.

Conflict of interest

None to declare.

.

Author details

Zeynep Özdemir and Mehmet Abdullah Alagöz
Faculty of Pharmacy, Department of Pharmaceutical Chemistry, İnönü University,
Malatya, Turkey

*Address all correspondence to: zeynep.bulut@inonu.edu.tr

IntechOpen

References

[1] Snell R. The Autonomic nervous system. In: Clinical Neuroanatomy. 7th ed. Philadelphia: Lippincott Publishers; 2010. pp. 120-125

[2] Lantsova VB, Sepp EK, Kozlovsky AS. Role sympathetic autonomic nervous system in the regulation of immune response during myasthenia. Bulletin of Experimental Biology and Medicine. 2011;**151**(3):353-355. DOI: 10.1007/s10517-011-1328-6

[3] Lemke T, Williams DA, Roche VF, Zito SW. Foye's Principles of Medicinal Chemistry. Philadelphia: Lippincott Williams & Wilkins; 2008. pp. 309-339

[4] Akyüz G, Akdeniz-Leblebiciler M. Anatomy and assessment of the autonomic nervous system. Turkish Journal of Physical Medicine and Rehabilitation. 2012;**58**(Suppl 1):1-5

[5] Mehndiratta MM, Pandey S, Kuntzer T. Acetylcholinesterase inhibitor treatment for myasthenia gravis. Cochrane Database of Systematic Reviews. 2011;**2**:CD006986. DOI: 10.1002/14651858.CD006986

[6] Drachman DB. Myasthenia gravis; review article in medical progress. The New England Journal of Medicine. 1994;**330**(25):1797-1810. DOI: 10.1056/NEJM199406233302507

[7] Meriggioli MN, Sheng JR, Li L, Prabhakar BS. Strategies for treating autoimmunity: Novel insights from experimental myasthenia gravis. Annals of the New York Academy of Sciences. 2008;**1132**:276-282. DOI: 10.1196/annals.1405.02

[8] Goodman Gilman A, Hardman JG, Limbird LE. Goodman & Gilman's The Pharmacological Basis of Therapeutics. 11th ed. New York: McGraw-Hill Medical Publishing Division; 2001. pp. 201

[9] Guyton AC, Hall JE. Medical Physiology. 11th ed. Vol. 87-89. Philadelphia, Pennsylvania: Elsevier Saunders; 2000. p. 751

[10] Zisimopoulou P, Lagoumintzis G, Poulas K, Tzartos SJ. Antigen-specific apheresis of human anti-acetylcholine receptor autoantibodies from myasthenia gravis patients' sera using *Escherichia coli*-expressed receptor domains. Journal of Neuroimmunology. 2008;**200**:133-141. DOI: 10.1016/j.jneuroim.2008.06.002

[11] Colovic MB, Krstic DZ, Lazarevic-Pasti TD, Bondzic AM, Vasic VM. Acetylcholinesterase inhibitors: pharmacology and toxicology. Current Neuropharmacology. 2013;**11**(3):315-335. DOI: 10.2174/1570159X11311030006

[12] Chatonnet A, Lockridge O. Comparison of butyrylcholinesterase and acetylcholinesterase. The Biochemical Journal. 1989;**260**(3):625-634

[13] Cheung J, Rudolph MJ, Burshteyn F, Cassidy MS, Gary EN, Love J, et al. Structures of human acetylcholinesterase in complex with pharmacologically important ligands. Journal of Medicinal Chemistry. 2012;**55**:10282-10286. DOI: 10.1021/jm300871x

[14] Dvir H, Silman I, Harel M, Rosenberry TL, Sussmana JL. Acetylcholinesterase: From 3D structure to function. Chemico-Biological Interactions. 2010;**187**: 10-22. DOI: 10.1016/j.cbi.2010.01.042

[15] Anand P, Singh P. A review on cholinesterase inhibitors for Alzheimer's disease. Archives of Pharmacal Research. 2013;**36**:375-399. DOI: 10.1007/s12272-013-0036-3

[16] Bourne Y, Taylor P, Radić Z, Marchot P. Structural insights into ligand interactions at the acetylcholinesterase peripheral anionic site. The EMBO Journal. 2003;**22**:1-12

[17] Changeux JP. Responses of acetylcholinesterase from Torpedo marmorata to salts and curarizing drugs. Molecular Pharmacology. 1966;**2**:369-392

[18] Pappano AJ. Cholinoceptor-activating & cholinesterase-inhibiting drugs. In: Katzung BG, Master SB, Trevor AJ, editors. Basic & Clinical Pharmacology. 12th ed. New York: McGraw-Hill Medical Publishing Division; 2012. p. 97

[19] Triggle DJ, Mitchell JM, Filler R. The pharmacology of physostigmine. CNS Drug Reviews. 2006;**4**(2):87-136. DOI: 10.1111/j.1527-3458.1998.tb00059.x

[20] Kelle İ. The effects of anticholinesterase drugs on bethanechol-induced contractile responses in rat ileum smooth muscle. Dicle Medical Journal. 2007;**34**(3):155-163

[21] Brenner T, Hamra-Amitay Y, Evron T, Boneva N, Seidman S, Soreq H. The role of readthrough acetylcholinesterase in the pathophysiology of myasthenia gravis. The FASEB Journal. 2003;**17**:214-222

[22] Sun C, Meng F, Li Y, Jin Q, Li H, Li F. Antigen-specific immunoadsorption of antiacetylcholine receptor antibodies from sera of patients with myastenia gravis. Artificial Cells, Blood Substitutes, and Immobilization Biotechnology. 2010;**38**(2):99-102. DOI: 10.3109/10731191003634778

[23] Strelnik AD, Petukhov AS, Zueva IV, Zobov VV, Petrov KA, Nikolsky EE, et al. Novel potent pyridoxine-based inhibitors of AChE and BChE, structural analogs of pyridostigmine, with improved in vivo safety profile. Bioorganic & Medicinal Chemistry Letters. 2016;**26**(16):4092-4094. DOI: 10.1016/j.bmcl.2016.06.070

[24] Amancio GCS, Grabe-Guimarãesa A, Haikel D, Moreau J, Barcellos NMS, Lacampagne A, et al. Effect of pyridostigmine on in vivo and in vitro respiratory muscle of mdx mice. Respiratory Physiology & Neurobiology. 2017;**243**:107-114. DOI: 10.1016/j.resp.2017.06.001

[25] Machado-Alba JE, Calvo-Torres LF, Avira-Mendoza A, Mejia-Velez CA. Prescription profile of pyridostigmine use in a population of patients with myasthenia gravis. Muscle & Nerve. 2017;**56**:1041-1046. DOI: 10.1002/mus.25625

[26] Lorke DE, Petroianu GA. Reversible cholinesterase inhibitors as pretreatment for exposure to organophosphates. A review. Journal of Applied Toxicology. 2018:1-16. DOI: 10.1002/jat.3662

[27] Hegazy N, Demirel M, Yazan Y. Preparation and in vitro evaluation of pyridostigmine bromide microparticles. International Journal of Pharmaceutics. 2002;**242**:171-174

[28] Petrov KA, Kharlamova AD, Lenina OA, Nurtdinov AR, Sitdykova ME, Ilyin VI, et al. Specific inhibition of acetylcholinesterase as an approach to decrease muscarinic side effects during myasthenia gravis treatment. Scientific Reports. 2018;**8**:304. DOI: 10.1038/s41598-017-18307-9

[29] Schmid O. Bis-Carbamic Acid Ester Compounds, and A Process of Making Same. U.S. Patent 2789981;1957

[30] Obara K, Chino D, Tanaka Y. Long-lasting inhibitory effects of distigmine on recombin-ant human acetylcholinesterase activity. Biological & Pharmaceutical

Bulletin. 2017;**40**:1739-1746. DOI:
10.1248/bpb.b17-00351

[31] Churchill-Davidson HC, Christie
TH. The diagnosis of neuromuscular
block in man. British Journal of
Anaesthesia. 1959;**31**:290-301

[32] Kent NB, Liang SS, Phillips S, Smith
NA, Khandkar C, Eikermann M, et al.
Therapeutic doses of neostigmine,
depolarising neuromuscular blockade
and muscle weakness in awake
volunteers: adouble-blind, placebo-
controlled, randomized volunteer study.
Anaesthesia. 2018;**73**:1079-1089. DOI:
10.1111/anae.14386

[33] Komloov M, Musilek K, Horova A,
Holas O, Dohnal V, Gunn-Moore F,
et al. Preparation, in vitro screening and
molecular modelling of symmetrical
bis-quinolinium cholinesterase
inhibitors—implications for early
Myasthenia gravis treatment.
Bioorganic & Medicinal Chemistry
Letters. 2011;**21**:2505-2509. DOI:
10.1016/j.bmcl.2011.02.047

[34] Barber HE, Calvey TN, Muir KT,
Taylor K. The effect of edrophonium
on erythrocyte acetylcholinesterase
and neuromuscular function in
the rat. British Journal of Clinical
Pharmacology. 2012;**56**(1):93-99

[35] Gold R, Schneider-Gold C. Current
and future standards in treatment of
myasthenia gravis. Neurotherapeutics.
2008;**5**(4):535-541

[36] Ra P, Stalberg E.
Acetylcholinesterase inhibitors in
myasthenia gravis: to be or not to be?
Muscle & Nerve. 2009;**39**:724-728

[37] Musilek K, Komloova M, Holas O,
Hrabinova M, Pohanka M, Dohnal V,
et al. Preparation and *in vitro* screening
of symmetrical bis-isoquinolinium
cholinesterase inhibitors bearing
various connecting linkage–Implications
for early Myasthenia gravis

treatment. European Journal
of Medicinal Chemistry.
2011;**46**(2):811-818

[38] Yu QS, Holloway HW, Luo W, Lahiri
DK, Brossi A, Greig NH. Long-acting
anticholinesterases for myasthenia
gravis: Synthesis and activities of
quaternary phenylcarbamates of
neostigmine, pyridostigmine and
physostigmine. Bioorganic & Medicinal
Chemistry. 2010;**18**:4687-4693. DOI:
10.1016/j.bmc.2010.05.022

[39] Argov Z, McKee D, Agus S, Brawer
S, Shlomowitz N, Yoseph OB, et al.
Treatment of human myasthenia
gravis with oral antisense suppression
of acetylcholinesterase. Neurology.
2007;**69**:699-700. DOI: 10.1212/01.
wnl.0000267884.39468.7a

[40] Brus B, Kosak U, Turk S, Pislar
A, Coquelle N, Kos J, et al. Discovery,
biological evaluation, and crystal
structure of a novel nanomolar selective
butyrylcholinesterase inhibitor.
Journal of Medicinal Chemistry.
2014;**57**:8167-8179

[41] Angelini CI, Martignago S, Bisciglia
M. New treatments for myasthenia: A
focus on antisense oligonucleotides.
Drug Design, Development and
Therapy. 2013;**7**:13-17